MYplace

FOR BIBLE STUDY

Published by First Place for Health
Galveston, Texas, U.S.A.
www.firstplaceforhealth.com
Printed in the U.S.A.

ISBN: 978-1-942425-50-2

CONTENTS

MY PLACE FOR BIBLE STUDY
Grace for the Race

FOREWORD

I was introduced to First Place for Health in 1993 by my mother-in-law, who had great concern for the welfare of her grandchildren. I was overweight and overwrought! God used that first Bible study to start me on my journey to health, wellness, and a life of balance.

Our desire at First Place for Health is for you to begin that same journey. We want you to experience the freedom that comes from an intimate relationship with Jesus Christ and witness His love for you through reading your Bible and through prayer. To this end, we have designed each day's study (which will take about fifteen to twenty minutes to complete) to help you discover the deep truths of the Bible. Also included is a weekly Bible memory verse to help you hide God's Word in your heart. As you start focusing on these truths, God will begin a great work in you.

At the beginning of Jesus' ministry, when He was teaching from the book of Isaiah, He said to the people, "The Spirit of the Lord is on me, because he has anointed me to preach good news to the poor. He has sent me to proclaim freedom for the prisoners and recovery of sight for the blind, to release the oppressed, to proclaim the year of the Lord's favor" (Luke 4:18–19). Jesus came to set us free—whether that is from the chains of compulsivity, addiction, gluttony, overeating, under eating, or just plain unbelief. It is our prayer that He will bring freedom to your heart so you may experience abundant life.

God bless you as you begin this journey toward a life of liberty.

Vicki Heath, First Place for Health National Director

ABOUT THE AUTHOR

Christin Ditchfield is passionate about calling believers to a deeper life—a life that's found in a deeper relationship with Jesus Christ. For thirty-five years, as an author and conference speaker and syndicated radio host, she's been encouraging people who love Jesus, teaching them to walk with Him on a daily basis, so that they can experience a richer, more meaningful relationship with Him.

As a professional freelance writer, Christin has written dozens of best-selling gospel tracts and hundreds of articles, essays, and columns for national and international Christian magazines. She is the author of more than 80 books, including the First Place for Health studies A New Beginning, A Thankful Heart, Living for Christ, Walking by Faith, and Finding Your Victory.

For years First Place for Health has been an important part of Christin's health and wellness journey. In addition to writing our Bible studies, she has been a member, a group leader, both a participant and speaker at Wellness Week retreats, and speaker at our annual Summit conference.

Christin holds a bachelor's degree in Christian Leadership, a master's degree in Bible and theology, and a doctorate in spiritual formation. Her husband, Andrew Lazo, is an author, scholar, and Episcopal priest. They make their home in Winter Garden, Florida, where they encourage each other in health and wellness by walking together in their neighborhood and competing in fitness challenges with their family and friends. For more information about Christin and her ministry, visit her website at www.ChristinDitchfield.com.

ABOUT THE CONTRIBUTOR

Lisa Lewis, who provided the menus and recipes in this study, is the author of Healthy Happy Cooking. Lisa's cooking skills have been a part of First Place for Health wellness weeks and other events for many years. She provided recipes for seventeen of the First Place for Health Bible studies and is a contributing author in Better Together and Healthy Holiday Living. She partners with community networks, including the Real Food Project, to bring healthy cooking classes to underserved areas. She is dedicated to bringing people together around the dinner table with healthy, delicious meals that are easy to prepare. Lisa lives in Galveston and is married to John. They have three children: Tal, Hunter, and Harper. Visit www.healthyhappycook.com for more delicious inspiration.

INTRODUCTION

First Place for Health is a Christ-centered health program that emphasizes balance in the physical, mental, emotional, and spiritual areas of life. The First Place for Health program is meant to be a daily process. As we learn to keep Christ first in our lives, we will find that He is the One who satisfies our hunger and our every need.

This Bible study is designed to be used in conjunction with the First Place for Health program but can be beneficial for anyone interested in obtaining a balanced lifestyle. The Bible study has been created in a seven-day format, with the last two days reserved for reflection on the material studied. Keep in mind that the ultimate goal of studying the Bible is not only for knowledge but also for application and a changed life. Don't feel anxious if you can't seem to find the correct answer. Many times, the Word will speak differently to different people, depending on where they are in their walk with God and the season of life they are experiencing. Be prepared to discuss with your fellow First Place for Health members what you learned that week through your study.

There are some additional components included with this study that will be helpful as you pursue the goal of giving Christ first place in every area of your life:

○ **Leader Discussion Guide:** This discussion guide is provided to help the First Place for Health leader guide a group through this Bible study. It includes ideas for facilitating a First Place for Health class discussion for each week of the Bible study.

○ **Jump Start Recipes:** There are seven days of recipes--breakfast, lunch and dinner-- to get you started.

○ **Steps for Spiritual Growth:** This section will provide you with some basic tips for how to memorize Scripture and make it a part of your life, establish a quiet time with God each day, and share your faith with others..

○ **First Place for Health Member Survey:** Fill this out and bring it to your first meeting. This information will help your leader know your interests and talents.

○ **Personal Weight and Measurement Record:** Use this form to keep a record of your weight loss. Record any loss or gain on the chart after the weigh-in at each week's meeting.

○ **Weekly Prayer Partner Forms:** Fill out this form before class and place it into a basket during the class meeting. After class, you will draw out a prayer request form, and this will be your prayer partner for the week. Try to call or email the person sometime before the next class meeting to encourage that person.

○ **100-Mile Club:** A worthy goal we encourage is for you to complete 100 miles of exercise during your time in First Place for Health. There are many activities listed on the 100-mile club pages at the back of this book that count toward your goal of 100 miles and a handy tracker to track your miles.

○ **Live It Trackers:** Your Live It Tracker is to be completed at home and turned in to your leader at your weekly First Place for Health meeting. The Tracker is designed to help you practice mindfulness and stay accountable with regard to your eating and exercise habits.

WEEK ONE: GRACE TO SAY YES

SCRIPTURE MEMORY VERSE

All athletes are disciplined in their training. They do it to win a prize that will fade away, but we do it for an eternal prize. 1 Corinthians 9:25

Can I tell you something? I have never thought of myself as an athlete. I don't have an athletic build. I don't have any of the natural talent, ability, coordination, or skill that it takes to compete in any physical activity—on any level. I don't even have the inclination. Sports are just not my thing.

But the Bible tells me that I have a body that is "fearfully and wonderfully made" (Psalm 139:14 NIV), created by God, in whom I live and move and have my being (Acts 17:28). I know I need to "move it or lose it." I need to take good care of this body I've been blessed with, even if I'm not always at peace with it. And I do like bling—which is how I came to sign up to walk my first half-marathon.

I was actually looking for a 5k (3.1 miles), a physical fitness challenge with a specific deadline that would motivate me to exercise more as part of my health and wellness journey. I just couldn't find one in my area with dates and times that worked for me.[1]

I did, however, find a half-marathon—13.1 miles—with a course that ran through a magical kingdom not far from where I lived, a race in which participants dressed up in costume as their favorite fairy tale characters—many in sparkly tutus and tiaras—and every participant received a gorgeous finisher medal, in addition to a cute t-shirt. I've always said, "If I'm going to exercise, I want a medal for it."

So, with very little idea of what I was getting myself into, and before I could talk myself out of it, I took a deep breath, registered, and began an adventure I'm still on today, fifteen years later.

I was only going to do that one race. In fact, it's the only way I finished the last three miles, telling myself over and over, "I NEVER have to do this again."

Now I have a rack on my wall for all the medals I've earned—5Ks, 10Ks, and to date, seven half-marathons. My younger self would be absolutely astounded.

With all that, I still haven't become an elite athlete. Or even a runner. (I walked every one of those races.) I don't race for the joy of racing itself. But I do love the motivation it gives me to keep up with my fitness routines. And I do love having done it—the sense of accomplishment. (I love the medals!) But more than anything, I love what I've learned in the process.

I now get why in Scripture the Apostle Paul repeatedly compared our spiritual life, the life of faith, to a race. In so many ways this life is like an epic race—and it's a marathon, not a sprint. We need grace to go the distance—grace and strength and courage and faith. Discipline and determination. Hope and patience and peace.

The good news is that God promises to give us all of these things—and so much more. He promises us His presence. He says He will be with us every step of the way. And He promises that one day, we WILL cross the finish line in victory.

The prize—the reward He has in store for us—is so much greater and will last so much longer than a t-shirt or a medal: "No eye has seen, no ear has heard, and no mind has imagined what God has prepared for those who love Him" (1 Corinthians 2:9). But God has given us all kinds of amazing hints.

Over the next eight weeks I'm going to share with you some of the things that I have learned and am still learning about this grace-filled race. We'll explore many powerful truths from Scripture that we can apply to our health and wellness journey and to every other challenge, obstacle, or adventure we face.

Because whether or not you see yourself as an athlete, whether or not you are physically able to take even a single step, you, too, are running the race of faith—daily.

Together let's "run to win!" (1 Corinthians 9:24).

—— DAY 1: SIGNING UP

God, thank You for calling me to this adventure, this journey, this race of faith. Thank You for Your goodness, Your love, Your mercy and grace.

Look up Isaiah 48:17. How does God describe Himself?

_____

_____

_____

How did He lead you to First Place for Health and this study?

_____

_____

_____

Why did you say "Yes!" and sign up for this? What's your "why"—your motivation or inspiration?

_____

_____

_____

What do you hope for and pray?

_____

_____

_____

What makes you anxious, worried, or afraid?

_____

_____

_____

In _Life-Giving Choices_, author Lucinda Secrest McDowell asks, "Is God calling you to move forward into the unknown? . . . Truth is, life is ever so much easier when we just sit on the couch. When we keep doing the same thing over and over again getting the same results. But who wants to live a life where nothing ever changes? Why not take a risk, when we know we have the King of the universe on our side?"[2]

Read Isaiah 43:1-3a. What does God say?

_____

_____

_____

In the Amplified Bible Hebrews 13:5b reminds us: "For He has said, 'I will never [under any circumstances] desert you [nor give you up nor leave you without support, nor will I in any degree leave you helpless], nor will I forsake you or let you down or relax my hold on you [assuredly not]!'"

How do these verses reassure your heart today?

_____

_____

_____

Lord, give me the courage and strength to "get off the couch"—physically, mentally, emotionally, and spiritually—today. Help me remember that You will be with me, every step of the way. Amen.

—— DAY 2: STUDYING UP

God, please give me a glimpse of where we are going –help me to see why You have chosen me, where You are leading me, and who You are calling me to be.

When you sign up for a race, you're given a map of the course—a big-picture view of where the road will take you. Let's look at the race of faith this way. Begin by reading Galatians 1:15, Ephesians 1:4-6, and 2 Timothy 1:9-10.

According to these verses, when did God first call Paul to join the race of faith? When did He call you?

_____

_____

_____

Why did God call Paul? Why did He call you? What was His big-picture plan or greater purpose? (There are several answers in these verses.)

_____

_____

_____

Read how The Message paraphrases Romans 8:29-30 and underline any words or phrases that resonate with you:

"God knew what he was doing from the very beginning. He decided from the out-set to shape the lives of those who love him along the same lines as the life of his Son. The Son stands first in the line of humanity he restored. We see the original and intended shape of our lives there in him. After God made that decision of what his children should be like, he followed it up by calling people by name. After he called them by name, he set them on a solid basis with himself. And then, after getting them established, he stayed with them to the end, gloriously completing what he had begun."

According to Ephesians 2:10, why did God do this? For what point or purpose?

What does your (physical, mental, emotional, spiritual) health and wellness have to do with this? Where do you see connections?

With decades of experience, former national director of First Place for Health Carole Lewis says,

I believe that lasting weight loss is dependent on our relationship with God. We can struggle and sweat all we want, and we can count calories and climb stairs, but until we learn to trust Him fully with our lives—until we rest in Him and let Him lead—we will never experience lasting success in this area.[3]

In *The Wellness Journey of a Lifetime*, our current national director Vicki Heath explains this is why First Place is not just about following a diet plan: "it's about developing a relationship with a person—Jesus Christ."[4] Our ultimate goal is to give Him first place in every area of our lives.

Our health and wellness matters because we matter to Him. He wants us to come to a place where we understand just how desperately He loves us and how desperately we need Him—in everything and for everything—because only He can help us live fully and freely as the glorious people of God He created us to be.

Jesus, thank You for everything! Thank You for loving me, saving me, and setting me free to live the life You have given to me, now and in eternity. Amen.

—— DAY 3: SAYING YES

Lord, open my eyes, my ears, my heart. Help me to respond to the invitation—the privilege and opportunity You have so generously offered me.

There comes a moment for each of us when—by God's grace—we decide that we're in, all in. We're saying, "Yes!" to Him. We're signing up and then showing up for whatever He has in store, trusting it will be a great adventure and that He will equip us, empower us, and be with us every step of the way.

When (and where and how) did you first hear and answer God's call? When did you first believe?

_____

_____

_____

What made you say "Yes!" to Him?

_____

_____

_____

To what has God called you in this season of your life—in this stretch of the race? What roles or responsibilities has He given you? What relationships? What ministry?

_____

_____

_____

Are you still saying "Yes!" to Him? If you are, in what ways? How? Why?

_____

_____

_____

If you haven't been, why not? What's getting in the way?

_____

_____

_____

Turn to Paul's prayer for believers in Ephesians 3:14-20. What does he ask God to give us? (See verses 17-18.)

_____

_____

_____

What does he want us to understand (verses 18-19)?

_____

_____

_____

Where can you find the power to say "Yes!" (and keep saying "Yes!") to God today? How can you be all that He has called you to be and do all that He has called you to do? How do you know this power is powerful enough (verse 20)?

_____

_____

_____

The Amplified Version of the Bible translates John 1:16 this way: For out of His fullness [the superabundance of His grace and truth] we have all received grace upon grace [spiritual blessing upon spiritual blessing, favor upon favor, and gift heaped upon gift].

How have you experienced this in your life to date? How does it motivate you or inspire you in your race of faith? What hope does it give you?

_____

_____

_____

God, here I am, signing up and showing up, saying "Yes!" to You for whatever You want to do in my heart and life today. Thank You for giving me grace upon grace. Amen.

—— DAY 4: STEPPING UP

God, I'm ready and willing to run my race today—at least, I want to be ready and willing. I'm willing to be made willing, and to take one step at a time by faith and by Your grace.

There are as many reasons to step up and sign up and show up for a race as there are runners—and just as many goals! Elite runners hope to win the race and set a record in the process. Others hope to be reasonably competitive and perhaps place in their age group. Some runners are challenging themselves to set their own record—their own personal best. Some are running to support other friends and family and keep them company. Some just want to cross the finish line and be able to say, "I did it!" And of course, some are there for the experience, the adventure of it. They want to have fun and make memories.

On Day 1 I asked you why you signed up for this First Place for Health study. Today, you're going to set some specific goals for this particular part of your race for the next eight weeks. Take a few moments to quiet your heart and mind. There's a reason the words on your mark and get set come before go!

Prayerfully consider where you are, physically, mentally, emotionally, and spiritually. Ask yourself—ask the Holy Spirit to show you--what's going well. What's not going well? What needs to change? Where is there room for growth or improvement? (You may want to answer these questions more fully in a separate notebook or journal.) Now choose a specific goal for each of the following areas or aspects of your life. Where do you want to be?

Physically:

_____

_____

_____

Mentally:

_____

_____

_____

Emotionally:

_____

_____

_____

Spiritually:

_____

_____

_____

Next list one specific step you can take—a change you can make—that will help you reach your goals. In other words, how will you get there?

Physically:

_____

_____

_____

Mentally:

_____

_____

_____

Emotionally:

_____

_____

_____

Spiritually:

_____
_____
_____

In Zechariah 4:10, we read: "Do not despise these small beginnings, for the Lord rejoices to see the work begin." How does this verse speak to you?

_____
_____
_____

Author and Bible teacher Jennifer Kennedy Dean made this powerful observation:

Choice by choice, act by act, decision by decision, obedience by obedience...a large life is made up of a whole lot of small . . . God has big plans for our lives. He intends for us 'exceedingly abundantly' more than we intend for ourselves. The big life He has for us is built small by small.[5]

Now turn to Joshua 1:9. What does this verse say? (You can copy it or write it in your own words, addressing your own life and the challenges you face.)

_____
_____
_____

Jesus, thank You for running this race with me. Thank You for running it before me—I know You know the way. I know You are the Way. I know You will help me today.

—— DAY 5: STARTING TODAY

God, help me to get off on the right foot this week. Show me where and how to start, what steps You want me to take. Be with me now, I pray.

Some people say they love running because it's simple. You don't need a lot of fancy equipment or an expensive membership to a gym or club. You can run (or walk) for exercise almost anywhere, even in your living room! That said, there are few basic things every runner needs—like a water bottle; loose, comfortable clothing; and a good, supportive pair of shoes. There are, of course, many other helpful tools—like a fitness tracker, a GPS app, music, and headphones.

So let's do a quick equipment check. What do you need to reach the goals you set yesterday? Any specific tools or supplies or resources you need to pull together? Is there any prep that needs to take place?

For instance—depending on your goals—you might do one or more of the following:

1. Download a fitness or nutrition app, or a Bible reading app, or a particular audio-book, or podcast series.
2. Create a playlist of great workout songs or praise songs.
3. Treat yourself to a new water bottle you promise yourself you will use.
4. Treat yourself to a new journal or pull out an old one that still has room.
5. Clear the laundry off the treadmill or exercise bike; track down those hand weights you've been using as doorstops. Or crawl under the bed and find your running shoes.
6. Ask a friend to be your walking buddy or join you at the gym; put a regular day and time on the calendar. (While you're at it, go ahead and note the dates of your First Place for Health sessions.)
7. Get rid of the junk food in the fridge and pantry and do a grocery shop.
8. Prep healthy snacks or grab-and-go meals ahead of time, so you're set for the week.
9. Take your measurements or do a basic fitness test, so that when you track your progress, you have more data than the number on the scale to note progress. (If numbers can be an issue for you, follow the example of one nutrition coach, who checks her fit with what she calls her "honesty pants.")
10. Set some kind of reminders (for whatever you want to remember) on your phone — or use sticky notes.
11. Sign up for a class—exercise, cooking, nutrition—or any kind of creative activity that helps you reach one of your physical, mental, emotional, or spiritual goals.

Your prep list

Let's go big-picture again, thinking about our race of faith, and look up Peter's prayer for believers in 2 Peter 1:2-4. What does Peter pray that God will give us?

_____

_____

_____

According to these verses, what has God already given us (verses 3-4)?

_____

_____

_____

How do we receive these gifts (verses 2-3)?

_____

_____

_____

How do these gifts help us (verse 4)?

_____

_____

_____

As we think about the goals we've set and what it will take to get there, what does Proverbs 3:5-6 remind us? (You can copy the reference here, write it in your own words, or look it up in a different translation.)

_____

_____

_____

What did the psalmist testify in Psalm 30:2?

_____

_____

_____

As you reflect on these verses, write your own prayer in the space below.

_____

_____

_____

Thank You, Lord, for all that You have promised me, all that You have provided for me. Thank You for hearing and answering my prayers.

—— DAY 6: REFLECTION AND APPLICATION
Lord, like the psalmist, I run in the path of Your commands, for You have set my heart free. Help me to run faithfully, persistently, courageously, and joyfully!

When you enter a race, you're given a bib to pin to the front of your shirt—essentially a large identifying number that sets you apart from the cheering fans in the crowd and the cadre of volunteers and race officials. Your bib identifies you as a competitor and says you belong on the course with all of the other athletes.

Take a few moments right now to design your own race bib for the next eight weeks in the figure below.

- In the border across the top, name this race something meaningful to you (or just use the name of this study).
- In the middle, give yourself a big, bold number, anywhere from 3-7 digits in length. (You might choose a significant date or the reference of a favorite Scripture.)
- Under the number write your first name in capital letters.
- In the border across the bottom, write a tagline or slogan—a short motivational phrase that inspires you, like "You got this!" or "Running to win!"
- Add some color, texture, and/or an image (like running shoes or a trophy, for example) to your design.

Different runners use different approaches, different training programs, and different strategies to prepare for and run their race. Listen to Paul's strategy for the race of faith in 1 Corinthians 9:24-25, as paraphrased in The Voice:

We all know that when there's a race, all the runners bolt for the finish line, but only one will take the prize. When you run, run for the prize! Athletes in training are *very strict with themselves, exercising self-control over desires, and for what?* For a wreath that soon withers *or is crushed or simply forgotten.* That is not our race. We run for the crown that we will wear for eternity.

So I don't run aimlessly. *I don't let my eyes drift off the finish line.* When I box, I don't throw punches in the air. I discipline my body and make it my slave so that after *all this,* after I have brought the gospel to others, I will still be qualified to *win the prize.*

Here's how Pastor Eugene Peterson paraphrased this same passage in The Message:

You've all been to the stadium and seen the athletes race. Everyone runs; one wins. Run to win. All good athletes train hard. They do it for a gold medal that tarnishes and fades. You're after one that's gold eternally.

I don't know about you, but I'm running hard for the finish line. I'm giving it everything I've got. No lazy living for me! I'm staying alert and in top condition. I'm not going to get caught napping, telling everyone else all about it and then missing out myself.

Using these verses as an example, describe your own motivation, inspiration, and focus. Write your race strategy in the space below. (Think of it like a mission, purpose, or passion statement.) It can be specific to your participation in First Place for Health or encompass your overall approach to the greater race of faith:

Lord, let all that I am, all that I do and say —and especially the way that I run this race—bring glory and honor to You today. Amen.

—— DAY 7: REFLECTION AND APPLICATION
Thank You, God, for all that You are doing in my heart and life today. Thank You for bringing me to this place and moment in time when I can experience Your goodness and grace.

Write this week's memory verse:

_____

_____

_____

Race Notes & Grace Notes

Where have you found grace for the race this week? How did you make progress or take positive steps in the right direction?

_____

_____

_____

Where did you struggle or stumble? What obstacles did you face?

_____

_____

_____

What have you learned that you want to take with you, going forward?

_____

_____

_____

What do you want to let go of or leave behind?

_____

_____

_____

What other glimpses of grace —grace upon grace—has God given you this week?

_____

_____

_____

"I do not at all understand the mystery of grace—only that it meets us where we are
but does not leave us where it found us."
—Anne Lamott

Lord Jesus, lead me on today—lead me to greater hope, greater trust, greater faith.
With every step, help me to grow in the knowledge of Your grace. Amen.

End Notes

1. First Place for Health now hosts its own virtual fitness challenges you can join at www.myplacetorace.com.

2. Lucinda Secrest McDowell, Life-Giving Choices: 60 Days to What Matters Most (Birmingham AL: New Hope Publishers, 2019), 17.

3. Carole Lewis with Marcus Brotherton, First Place 4 Health: Discover a New Way to Healthy Living (Ventura CA: Regal Books, 2008), 93.

4. Vicki Heath, The Wellness Journey of a Lifetime (Galveston TX: First Place 4 Health, 2015), 23.

5. Jennifer Kennedy Dean, The Power of Small: Think Small to Live Large, (Birmingham AL: New Hope Publishers, 2011), 13-14.

WEEK TWO: GRACE TO SAY NO

SCRIPTURE MEMORY VERSE

Therefore, since we are surrounded by such a huge crowd of witnesses to the life of faith, let us strip off every weight that slows us down, especially the sin that so easily trips us up. And let us run with endurance the race God has set before us.
Hebrews 12:1

More than once, I've said "no" to the cozy comfort of my nice, warm hotel bed—and several hours more of much-needed sleep—so I could drag myself out to the curb to catch a 3 a.m. shuttle to the starting line of a race that suddenly seemed like a ridiculously crazy idea.

The bigger the race, the earlier you have to arrive because it takes time to line up thousands of people. You often end up standing there on the concrete, shivering in the cold for two or three hours before the 5 a.m. or 6 a.m. start time.

Some people wear hoodies or wrap themselves in thermal blankets (or trash bags); others huddle together chatting, munching on snacks, and taking selfies, occasionally stepping away to stretch or jump up and down or jog in place to stay warm.

If you've ever done one of these events, you know that once the race begins, the side of the road becomes a massive debris field. It's covered in cast-off blankets, jackets, hats and gloves, drawstring backpacks, empty food wrappers and water bottles, and unraveled ace bandages. As the race goes on, you'll see more layers being shed, and bits of costume accessories—ribbons, headbands, tutus, fairy wings—that looked super-cute in those selfies, but turned out not to be so comfortable for running long distance.

That's what I picture now when I read this week's Scripture Memory Verse—runners I've seen stripping off everything that's suddenly become too hot, too heavy, too tight, or too itchy—anything that's weighing them down or keeping them from running freely. They've worked too hard and trained too long to let anything unnecessary distract them or trip them up now. They've got their eyes on the prize—they want to cross that finish line.

This is how we want to be! Whether we're talking about our health and wellness race or our greater (big picture) race of faith, we want to "just say no" and let go of anything that will keep us from victory.

Titus 2:11-14 (NIV) reminds us,

> For the grace of God has appeared that offers salvation to all people. It teaches us to say "No" to ungodliness and worldly passions, and to live self-controlled, upright and godly lives in this present age, while we wait for the blessed hope—the appearing of the glory of our great God and Savior, Jesus Christ, who gave Himself for us to redeem us from all wickedness and to purify for himself a people that are his very own, eager to do what is good.

Let's look at some things we want to say "no" to this week.

—— DAY 1: NO TO SIN

Jesus, thank You for Your blood, which was shed for me. Thank You for dying on the cross to set me free from the power of sin. Help me to walk in that freedom and run in that freedom today.

Our memory verse this week describes "sin that so easily trips us up." Other Bible translations use phrases like "so easily entangles," "deftly and cleverly clings to us," "catches us," "ensnares us," "slackens our pace," or "holds us so tight."

Once a friend texted to ask how my "race" was going—how I was doing with my healthy eating. I thought about all the temptation I'd been giving in to, and responded with a graphic of someone face-planting.

How is your race going right now? What kind of graphic would you use?

If you had to name one or two, what sins seem to be the biggest obstacles for you? What's been slowing you down, tripping you up, or sending you sprawling spiritually?

_____

_____

_____

Remember that eating a slice of cake or skipping a workout is NOT in and of itself sin—it may simply not be the best choice. For some it may even be unwise or unhealthy. (But in some cases, it could actually be a GOOD choice for you.)

It MAY be sinful if it's rooted in a deeper heart issue—a symptom of what Scripture clearly identifies as sin (like greed, lust, idolatry, laziness, complacency, or disobedience to or rebellion against God).

In Week 7, we'll talk a lot more about sin and temptation, but for now let's look at a few key verses that can help us see sin for what it is and find the grace to "just say no."

What does Romans 5:6-11 remind us?

_____

_____

_____

What does Romans 6:12-14 urge us to do?

_____

_____

_____

What does Romans 8:5-7 teach us?

_____

_____

_____

Look up Psalm 79:9. Where did the psalmist turn when he found sin had entangled him again?

_____

_____

_____

What does God say in Isaiah 1:18?

_____

_____

_____

In Psalm 65:1-3 for what does the psalmist praise God?

_____

_____

_____

How might remembering what God has done for you and filling your mouth with His praise help you say "no" to sin today?

_____

_____

_____

Thank You, Jesus! Your grace amazes me. Thank You for forgiveness and fresh starts, new mornings and new mercies. Thank You for the power to say "no" to sin and "yes" to You.

—— DAY 2: NO TO LESSER THINGS

Lord, direct my steps today. Lead me and guide me in every choice that I make. Help me to run this race with focus, courage, and determination.

It's important to remember that every time we say "yes" to something, we're saying "no" to something else. You and I don't have unlimited resources—unlimited time, energy, and focus. We can only take on so many tasks, so many responsibilities, so many projects at any given time. We can only maintain so many relationships.

That's why we need God's grace to learn how and when (and to what and to whom) we should say "no." It's why we need to constantly reexamine our priorities in light of our goals and God's calling on our lives in this particular season of our lives. We need to look at how we choose to spend our time and energy and prayerfully consider what we might need to do differently. We need the Holy Spirit's help to identify things in our lives that are not necessarily bad—and may even be good at the right time for the right person—but are not good for us right now . . . things that may overburden us, weigh us down, drain our time or energy, or become a hindrance or distraction. As the saying goes, "Good things become bad when they keep us from the best!"

Look up 1 Corinthians 10:23. What expression did Paul use that can be helpful for us here?

_____

_____

_____

Read Luke 10:38-42. What did Martha think was the problem?

_____

_____

_____

What did Jesus identify as the real problem? Why was this a problem for this woman in this situation?

_____

_____

_____

Note that Jesus didn't have anything against generous hospitality. On the contrary, in the Gospels we see Him rebuke ungenerous hosts and warn of the dangers of being short-sighted, unwise, and unprepared. He also both modeled and affirmed positive examples (such as when He washed His disciples' feet and when He blessed the woman who washed His feet with her tears).

How did He describe Mary's choice in this particular time and place? Why?

_____

_____

_____

What does Ecclesiastes 3:1-8 remind us?

_____

_____

_____

How would you describe the time and season you find yourself in?

_____

_____

_____

Why is God calling you to prioritize your health and wellness?

_____

_____

_____

What does that mean? What does it look like for you?

_____

_____

_____

What might you need to say "no" to, so that you can make healthier choices?

_____

_____

_____

In the words of the old hymn,

Rise up, O saints of God!
Have done with lesser things;
give heart and soul and mind and strength
to serve the King of kings.[1]

God, show me Your priorities for me. Help me to say "no" to—or let go of—anything that would keep me from accomplishing these things, for Your Kingdom and Your glory.

—— DAY 3: NO TO DOUBT AND DOUBLE-MINDEDNESS

Lord, help me to trust You and the path You have set before me and not second-guess every step I take. Give me strength, resolve, and determination today. I pray this in Jesus's Name.

Read James 1:5-8 and Ephesians 4:14. What spiritual problem do these verses address?

_____

_____

_____

What did Jesus say about being uncommitted or double-minded in Luke 9:62?

_____

_____

_____

In 1 Corinthians 15:58 what does God call us to do or be instead?

_____

_____

_____

In *Your Future Self Will Thank You: Secrets to Self-Control from the Bible and Brain Science*, Drew Dyck writes about research that shows how many decisions we make on a daily basis and how much energy it takes us to make those decisions, leaving us with less energy (or willpower) to make more decisions, to make and keep making healthy choices, and to resist temptation.

What makes our struggle even worse is we keep remaking our decisions—changing our minds over and over again about, for example, what is or isn't "on plan," what we will or won't eat today, and when or how we will exercise.

Dyck writes that willpower is "a finite resource. Expend enough willpower by tackling difficult tasks or resisting temptation and eventually your willpower reserves will run dry. You can build your willpower. You can be strategic about how you use it.

But ultimately you only have so much. That's where habits help. Once a behavior becomes encoded as a habit, it no longer requires effort."[2]

Science and the Bible agree, Dyck says, that it's so much better to make small, consistent, positive changes over time (one at a time) day after day. These positive changes become good habits and healthy routines—which means we do them automatically, without thinking (or rethinking) about them. And then of course, we have more energy or willpower for whatever specific challenges we're facing on any given day.

Dyck adds, "When I look back at many of my attempts to get healthier or practice a spiritual discipline, I'm struck by how often I've given up after a week or two. Often we don't even realize how close we come to that magical threshold where the behavior becomes second nature. Now, when I'm trying to create a new habit, I'm conscious of pushing through to that point. It's encouraging to know that the behavior will become more automatic as I go, demanding less and less effort over time."[3]

What's one healthy habit (physically, mentally, emotionally, or spiritually) that is already a part of your routine? When did you establish this habit? How has it benefited you?

_____

_____

_____

What's one thing you'd like to make a new habit or a routine?

_____

_____

How will you commit yourself to this new habit or routine? What steps will you take and when? What will you say "no" to, so that you can say "yes" to this?

_____

_____

_____

What encouragement do you find in Psalm 37:5-6?

_____

_____

_____

Thank You, Jesus, for giving me wisdom in my decision-making today. Please give me healthy resolve, too—the strength to follow through. Let my obedience become a holy habit that glorifies You.

—— DAY 4: NO TO NEGATIVITY
God, give me a cheerful heart today. Help me to rejoice in You, in all the good things You do, and in all the good things You've given me to do.

We don't have to eat right and exercise—we get to partner with God in healthy living, in caring for the bodies He has given us. We don't have to say "no" to "everything that hinders and the sin that so easily entangles." We get to say "no," because Jesus shed His blood to give us the freedom and the power to do so! (See Romans 6:4-7.) We get to say "yes" to Him! We get to obey Him with our hearts full of love and gratitude instead of obeying sin.

How does Jude 16 describe people who are still in bondage to sin?

_____

_____

_____

What does 1 Thessalonians 5:16-18 tell us we should do or be instead?

_____

_____

_____

What does Philippians 2:14-15 tell us to do and not to do—to be and not to be?

_____

_____

_____

Now look up Colossians 3:16-17. What can we do to have a happy heart? A positive outlook or attitude? (There are five things.)

1. _____

2. _____

3. _____

4. _____

5. _____

Let's practice this! Choose three things that you often find yourself grumpy or grumbling about—health and wellness things or anything really—and turn these "have to's" into "get to's." Sometimes this kind of exercise is called "reframing," because it helps us see things differently.

I've done one of my own for you:

Ugh! I HAVE to make six trips up the stairs with all this laundry.

Thank You, Jesus, that I get to do this. This is one of the ways I get to show love for my family. Thank You for clothes to wear and the machines to launder them and thank You that my body will carry me up those stairs. It hasn't always. You have healed my broken bones and given me new strength and energy. Hallelujah!

That reminds me — I keep meaning to tell you: One of the reasons I enter these races I've been talking about is because I can . . . and I want to celebrate that! I live with chronic pain. I've had nine knee surgeries on the same knee—bone grafts and screws and joint replacement. In the middle of it all, I broke that same leg twice in one calendar year. When I add all the various weeks and months of recovery together, I can say I've spent three full years of my life on crutches. Believe me, being able to walk across a room with my arms full of laundry is a gift and a blessing!

Your turn:

I *have* to . . .

_____

I *get* to . . .

_____

I *have* to . . .

_____

I *get* to . . .

_____

I *have* to . . .

_____

I *get* to . . .

_____

How do you think having a "get to" perspective can help you run your race today?

_____
_____
_____

Thank You, Jesus, for the freedom to choose joy and gratitude. Thank You for all You have done for me and all You have given me. I love You. It's my pleasure to serve You.

—— DAY 5: NO TO LUST AND GREED

Lord, I have so much to be grateful for and so many reasons to be content with what You've given me. Help me to desire only You and Your good gifts, and nothing more.

In the introduction to this week, we read in Titus 2 that the grace of God helps us say "no" to "worldly passions." That's what we're talking about today: unhealthy or destructive desires that, left unchecked, would destroy us and everything we hold dear.

James 1:14-15 tells us, "Temptation comes from our own desires, which entice us and drag us away. These desires give birth to sinful actions. And when sin is allowed to grow, it gives birth to death."

So what are these desires? What else does the Bible tell us about where they come from? What else is the result?

Look up the following Scriptures and fill out the chart below:

Verses	Desire	Source	Result
Colossians 3:5-6			
1 John 2:15-17			
Mark 7:21-23			
Galatians 1:10			
Galatians 5:19-21			

What unhealthy desires are you aware of in your own life today? What do you battle?

_____

_____

_____

What does God want you to desire and be filled with instead? (See Galatians 5:22-23.)

_____

_____

_____

What does Galatians 5:24 tell us about those who belong to Christ?

_____

_____

_____

What does Galatians 5:25 urge us to do? Why?

_____

_____

_____

According to Philippians 2:13, how is this possible?

_____

_____

_____

What did the psalmist pray in Psalm 51:10?

_____

_____

_____

What is your prayer?

_____

_____

_____

God, change my heart today. Give me the desire to love You and serve You so much more than I do. Give me the desire to do good—to do what pleases You—and give me the power to obey.

—— DAY 6: REFLECTION AND APPLICATION

Thank You, Father, for Your tender love for me. Thank You for all the hope and help and strength You give me.

This week we've been talking about finding the grace to say "no" to anything and everything that would keep us from running to win. We battle all kinds of temptations, all kinds of unhealthy habits, attitudes, behaviors, and destructive desires that "wage war" against our souls (1 Peter 2:11). But we don't have to do it alone. Jesus promises to be with us and to help us, moment by moment.

In his book *Every Moment Holy*, author Douglas Kaine McKelvey offers "A Liturgy for One Battling a Destructive Desire."

Read through this prayer slowly—prayerfully—underlining any words or phrases that speak to you. Then read it again out loud, as a prayer from your heart to God's. Pray it and keep praying it, as often as you need to this week:

Jesus, here I am again, desiring a thing that were I to indulge in it would war against my own heart and the hearts of those I love. O Christ, rather let my life be thine! Take my desires. Let them be subsumed in still greater desire for You, until there remains no room for these lesser cravings.

In this moment I might choose to indulge a fleeting hunger, or I might choose to love you more. Faced with this temptation, I would rather choose you, Jesus—but I am weak. So be my strength. I am shadowed. Be my light. I am selfish. Unmake me now, and refashion my desires according to the better designs of your love.

Given the choice of shame or glory, let me choose glory. Given the choice of this moment or eternity, let me choose in this moment what is eternal. Given the choice of this easy pleasure or the harder road of the cross, give me grace to choose to follow you, knowing that there is nowhere apart from your presence where I might find the peace I long for, no lasting satisfaction apart from your reclamation of my heart.

Let me build then, my King, a beautiful thing by long obedience, by the steady progression of small choices that laid end to end will become like the stones of a pleasing path stretching to eternity and unto your welcoming arms, and unto the sound of your voice pronouncing the judgment:

Well done.[4]

What is God speaking to your heart today? What small choices is He asking you to make? How will you respond? Going forward, what will you say "yes" to? What will you say "no" to?

_____

_____

_____

God, my heart and my flesh may fail, but You are the strength of my heart and my portion forever. All my hope is in You.

—— DAY 7: REFLECTION AND APPLICATION

Lord, thank You for the grace to say "no" to "everything that hinders" and the grace to say "yes" — and keep saying "yes" — to You.

Write this week's memory verse:

_____

_____

_____

Race Notes & Grace Notes
Where have you found grace for the race" this week? Where did you make progress or take positive steps in the right direction?

_____

_____

_____

Where did you struggle or stumble? What obstacles did you face?

_____

_____

_____

What have you learned that you want to take with you, going forward?

_____

_____

_____

What do you want to let go of or leave behind?

_____

_____

_____

What other glimpses of grace —grace upon grace—has God given you this week?

_____

_____

_____

"God's grace is amazing! We're saved by grace—God's undeserved favor—and we live by grace, which is also God's power in our lives to do what we could never do in our own strength. And it's all because God is love, and He loves us unconditionally, constantly and completely."
—Joyce Meyer

God, give me the grace to remember Your great love for me. Help me to rest in that love, live in that love, and share that love with everyone I meet, as I run this race today. Amen.

End Notes

1. William P. Merrill. 1911. "Rise Up, O Saints of God," also published as "Rise Up, O Men of God." Public Domain.

2. Drew Dyck, Your Future Self Will Thank You: Secrets to Self-Control from the Bible and Brain Science, (Chicago: Moody Publishers, 2019), 97.

3. Drew Dyck, Your Future Self, 132.

4. Douglas Kaine McKelvey, Every Moment Holy, Volume 1 (Nashville: Rabbit Room Press, 2017),165-166. Used with permission.

WEEK THREE: GRACE TO HOLD ON

SCRIPTURE MEMORY VERSE

We do this by keeping our eyes on Jesus, the champion who initiates and perfects our faith. **Hebrews 12:2**

When I began training for my first half-marathon, I learned that the race had a pace requirement. I would have to be able to walk a fifteen-minute mile—well, actually, thirteen consecutive fifteen-minute miles—or risk being "swept" off the course. (The roads have to reopen eventually, and the staff and volunteers need to go home. They can't wait at the finish line all day!)

I was really, really worried I wouldn't be able to keep up. Terrified, honestly. But then I discovered that there were training programs developed by wise and experienced coaches that would help me and workout schedules I could follow to gradually increase both my speed and my endurance. The coaches had books, websites, and videos that answered common questions and provided encouragement and advice.

So I learned everything I could and laced up my shoes. And I went for a lot of walks, passing the miles by visualizing crossing the finish line—looking ahead, imagining how good it would feel to get there and how proud and excited I would be.

I did a lot of praying on those walks. Especially on days when it was really hot or really cold or I was really tired and didn't think I could make it to the end of my training walk, let alone the actual race.

"Lord Jesus, help me!"

In the First Place for Health Study *Training for Success,* Janet Holm McHenry points out that in any area of our life, any part of the race we're running, Jesus is the best coach—the best Personal Trainer—that any of us could ask for.

Depending on which Bible translation you read, Hebrews 12:2 calls Him "the champion," the "author and perfector" of our faith, "the pioneer and perfector," the "initiator and completer," "leader and finisher," the "leader and the source," or the "source and the goal," or the "originator and instructor." He's all these good things, and so much more.

Janet points out, "While He was (and is) fully God, He was also fully man during His 30-some years on this earth. In fact, Jesus faced the same kinds of temptations, disappointments, struggles, and hurts that we do today. Yet in spite of the challenges, His life was purposeful and victorious"[1]—and ours can be, too if we keep our eyes on Him.

Jesus knows better than we do what we're up against. He's already covered the terrain. He knows all the best training techniques and race day strategies. And He knows us—our strengths and our weaknesses, our temperaments and our personalities. He knows when (and how hard) to push us—when to challenge us, when to comfort us, and when to tell us to take a break.

He knows the perfect pace to set. In Matthew 11:28-30 in The Message, He says, in part, "Walk with me and work with me—watch how I do it. Learn the unforced rhythms of grace."

Author Pam Farrel writes, "Do you feel as if you're running out of steam, that you cannot endure any longer? Ask God to lift you up and give you renewed energy. God will send you what and who you need to hold on to the adventure He has planned for you."[2]

Look to Him. He will coach you and keep you company every step of the way.

—— DAY 1: HOLD ON TO WHO JESUS IS AND WHAT HE HAS DONE

Thank You, Jesus, for being here with me right now. Thank You for running this race before me and for running it with me today.

If you're going to trust Jesus as your Personal Trainer –if you're going to give him your heart and your life, as well as all your hopes and dreams and plans—you probably should be familiar with His bio and resume! It's a good idea to remember why you put yourself in His hands.

Read Colossians 1:9-22 and answer these questions: Who is Jesus? What has He done?

_____

_____

_____

What does Phlippians 2:5-11 add?

_____

_____

_____

What does Matthew 12:18-20 tell you about His coaching style?

_____

_____

_____

Why can we have confidence in Jesus, according to Matthew 12:21?

_____

_____

_____

Author Kendra Smiley writes that in Sunday school or children's church, kids often just shout "the all-purpose answer to any question": _Jesus!_ We should follow their example, Kendra says, because "no matter what is happening in your life or in your home today, Jesus is the answer."[3]

Where do you need His help as you run your race today?

_____

_____

_____

Remember who He is and call on Him. Ask Him for that help right now:

_____

_____

_____

Lauraine Snelling writes, "Let's all hang onto our Savior's hand and keep looking at His Face. Such glory and love shining unto and into us!"[4]

_____

_____

_____

Lord Jesus, I'm looking to You. I'm listening to You. I'm trusting You. You know the way that I take. So wherever You lead, I will follow. Whatever You say, I will obey.

—— DAY 2: HOLD ON TO WHAT IS TO COME

Jesus, please help me to see You—really see You –today. Keep getting my attention when it drifts. Keep lifting my gaze to Your beautiful face.

In Numbers 21 we learn of a time when God's people were rebelling against Him, complaining about how long and how hard their wilderness "training" was turning out to be. They didn't like the conditions. They didn't like the provisions. They didn't like or trust the way He was leading them. Then when they started getting bitten by poisonous snakes, they finally cried out to God to save them, and God told Moses to craft a bronze snake on a pole and hold it up high. Everyone who looked up at it would be instantly healed and saved.

In John 3:14-15, Jesus said that this was a real-life object lesson to point us to Him! One day He would be lifted up on the cross. And everyone who looked to Him would be saved. In the verse right after this one, He explains why:

For God so [greatly] loved and dearly prized the world, that He [even] gave His [One and] only begotten Son, so that whoever believes and trusts in Him [as Savior] shall not perish, but have eternal life. (John 3:16 AMP)

When did you first lift your eyes and look to Jesus this way?

_____

_____

_____

How are you looking to Him today?

_____

_____

_____

Psalm 123:2 says, "We keep looking to the LORD our God for his mercy, just as servants keep their eyes on their master, as a slave girl watches her mistress for the slightest signal." We could also say, "As athletes look to their coach or trainer!" Why do you think is it so important for us to keep our eyes on Him—to keep looking to Him and keep trusting Him?

_____

_____

_____

Author Jane Rubietta says sometimes we get busy with things that just don't matter in the light of eternity. When we finally look up,

> "We see those eyes. They beam with love and appreciation and a forever commitment. Jesus just waits to meet our eyes and pour into us His eternal affection. Do you see Him? Can you find His gaze? Do you see that brilliant smile break over His face—like the sunrise—and know: you are His, and He is crazy about you? And He is . . . just loving you? And there is no need to look anywhere else. Heaven has come to earth and you have a Lover who is dying to be with you."[5]

Why is this perspective so powerful—even life-changing? How can it help us run our race?

_____

_____

_____

What does each of the following verses tell us we are looking for?
Revelation 1:7 _____
Revelation 1:18 _____
Luke 12:37 _____
Romans 5:2 _____
2 Timothy 4:8 _____
Hebrews 13:14 _____
2 Peter 3:13 _____

In light of these truths, what can you let go of today? What will you hold on to?

_____

_____

_____

Jesus, when I get just a glimpse of how much You love me and when I catch a vision of who You really are, what You are doing, where You are leading, and what You have in store for me, such hope fills my heart! Thank You, Jesus. I love You.

—— DAY 3: HOLD ON TO WHAT HE HAS PROMISED

Lord Jesus, You are my Savior, my strength, and my song. I will praise You all day long with my whole heart!

Keeping our eyes on Jesus means remembering and holding on to who He is, what He has done, and what He has promised to do. This whole study is full of precious promises from His Word, promises we can cling to. Today let's look at a few of those promises more closely.

For what does the psalmist praise God in Psalm 103:1-5? (There are at least six things.)

What do we learn about Him in Psalm 84:11?

For what reason does Paul rejoice in Philippians 4:19?

What did the psalmist declare in Psalm 145:15?

What do we learn from Acts 17:24-25 and Psalm 107:9?

_____

_____

_____

Remember that in John 10:10, Jesus said He had come to give His people "a rich and satisfying life," a life full of "joy and abundance" (VOICE)—"real and eternal life, more and better life than they ever dreamed of" (MSG).

What did God promise in Psalm 81:10?

_____

_____

_____

What would all these promises say about the character of God?

_____

_____

_____

In her book *Full: Food, Jesus, and the Battle for Satisfaction,* Asheritah Ciuciu writes, "Life with Jesus is full: full of joy in His presence, full of the riches of His glory, full of comfort in sufferings, full of rejoicing in hardships, full of pleasures at His right hand, full of life in this world and the next . . . something that deeper and more satisfying than the most delicious feast."[6]

How have you experienced this in your own life? Can you think of a specific example?

_____

_____

_____

Where do you want or need to experience this?

_____

_____

_____

How can you connect all of this to the race you're running for greater health and wellness? How will it help you run your race today?

_____

_____

_____

Thank You, Jesus, for the many ways You promise to satisfy my hunger and meet all of my needs. Remind me to always run to You first.

—— DAY 4: HOLD ON TO WHAT WE'VE BEEN GIVEN

God, thank You for Your Word. Thank You for Your love. Thank You for Your kindness and goodness and mercy toward me. Thank You for leading the way and going before me into this day.

When we're in a difficult or challenging place---a tough part of the race—we often tell ourselves (and others) to "hold on" or "hang in there!" In other words, "Don't give up! Don't give in! It will get better. It's going to be okay."

Where do you need this reminder today?

_____

_____

_____

Let's look at some of the things the Scripture tells us to hold on to—and how and why. Look up each verse and jot down what it says about this:

Deuteronomy 11:22 _____

Romans 12:9 _____

Ephesians 6:16-17_____

Philippians 2:16_____

Philippians 3:16_____

1 Timothy 6:12 _____

Hebrews 4:14_____

Hebrews 6:18 _____

Revelation 3:11 _____

Look back over your notes. Choose one or two verses that speak to you. Whom or what do you need to hold on to? Why?

_____

_____

_____

How will this verse, this truth, help you run your race? How can you connect this to your health and wellness journey? What will it keep you from doing? What will it help you to do?

_____

_____

_____

_____

_____

If you can, take a few moments to listen to Rich Mullins's song "Bound to Come Some Trouble" (look it up on YouTube or your favorite music streaming service) or another song that encourages you to hold on.

_____

_____

_____

Thank You, Jesus, for giving me the strength to hold on to You today. Help me to hold on to every word You say, every promise You make. And help me keep my promises to You.

—— DAY 5: JESUS HOLDS ON, TOO

Lord, You are so strong and mighty, there's nothing that You can't do, nothing You can't carry, and nothing that can be snatched away from You. You are the safest place in all the world that I can run to.

Today we're going to take a look at who or what Jesus holds on to—just a few of the many people and things the Scripture says He's got in His hands—and what that means. Look up each verse and jot down what it says about this:

Psalm 3:3 _____

Psalm 18:48 _____

Psalm 37:24 _____

Psalm 63:8 _____

Psalm 95:4 _____

Isaiah 41:10 _____

Isaiah 62:3 _____

Colossians 1:17 _____

Colossians 2:19 _____

Revelation 1:18 _____

Look back over your notes. Choose one or two verses that speak to you. How is this truth a comfort or encouragement to you?

_____

_____

_____

How will this truth help you run your race today?

_____

_____

_____

While we're talking about being held, there's one more verse I'd like to share with you. I often use the imagery in this verse as I pray for myself and for those I love. Remember that in John 10:1-16 (and many other Scriptures) Jesus says He is our Good Shepherd and we are His sheep.

Here's what Isaiah 40:11 tells us: "He will feed His flock like a shepherd. He will carry the lambs in His arms, holding them close to His heart."

Turn this verse into a prayer for yourself today:

_____

_____

_____

Now pray it specifically for someone you love:

....

....

....

As I pray, I'm also encouraged by John 10:28-29, where Jesus says: "I give them eternal life, and they will never perish. No one can snatch them away from me, for my Father has given them to me, and He is more powerful than anyone else. No one can snatch them from the Father's hand."

Hebrews 13:5 (AMP) reminds us, "He has said, 'I will never [under any circumstances] desert you [nor give you up nor leave you without support, nor will I in any degree leave you helpless], nor will I forsake or let you down or relax my hold on you [assuredly not]!'"

How do these scriptures encourage you?

....

....

....

Sometimes in my journal I draw a hand (or print out a picture of one from an internet search) and write my name and the names of others across the palm, along with these Scriptures — and Isaiah 49:16, where God says, "See, I have written your name on the palms of My hands."

You might do something similar in the space below:

....

....

....

Jesus, You never forget me. You never abandon me or forsake me. While I'm holding on to You, You're holding on to me and to those who are precious to me. Thank You for keeping us safe in Your love.

—— DAY 6: REFLECTION AND APPLICATION

Thank You, God, for the grace to stay focused today. Thank You for the grace to hold on to what I know is true—Your love for me and my love for You.

A hundred years ago artist and missionary Lilias Trotter observed a little dandelion in a forest, looking positively radiant as it lifted its face to the sun. She started thinking about what happens to us when we turn our faces to the "Sun of Righteousness"--Jesus–and make Him our focus—how our lives are so beautifully transformed—transfigured. We shine with the light of His glory, and everything else fades away.

In a devotional essay she wrote, "Turn full your soul's vision to Jesus, and look and look at Him, and a strange dimness will come over all that is apart from Him."[7]

The psalmist prayed: "Turn my eyes from worthless things, and give me life through your word." (Psalm 119:37) He urges, "Search for the LORD and for his strength; continually seek him. Remember the wonders he has performed, his miracles..." (Psalm 105:4-5) "Those who look to him for help will be radiant with joy; no shadow of shame will darken their faces." (Psalm 34:4-5)

When Helen Lemmel heard Lilias Trotter's words, they touched her deeply. At the beginning of the twentieth century, Helen was a professional musician and singer-songwriter who performed at churches and in concert halls all over the country. She had experienced great success. She had also faced her share of heartache and pain, being widowed as a young woman and raising two children on her own. Helen had found love again and traveled the world with her second husband–only to be abandoned by him a few years into their marriage, when, in her late forties, she suddenly went blind. (Her husband said he just couldn't handle caring for a disabled wife.) Now in her fifties, she was alone and financially destitute.

Helen could have fallen into a deep spiritual darkness, consumed by grief over what she had lost or filled with fear over what the future would hold for her. But she knew who held her and her future. She would live the rest of her very long life—she lived to be 97—lifting her face to Jesus, looking to Him daily to be her provider and protector. She wrote Him nearly five hundred songs of praise, one of them inspired by Lilias's essay. You probably know it:

O soul are you weary and troubled
No light in the darkness you see
There's light for a look at the Savior
And life more abundant and free

Turn your eyes upon Jesus
Look full in His wonderful face
And the things of earth will grow strangely dim
In the light of His glory and grace.[8]

How have you been weary or troubled lately? What "things of earth" have been a distraction or discouragement to you?

_____

_____

_____

What does it mean to you to "turn your eyes upon Jesus"? How would you put it in your own words?

_____

_____

_____

On a very practical level, what can you do to keep Him your focus today? This week?

_____

_____

_____

What truths will you hold on to as you run your race?

_____

_____

_____

Thank You, Jesus, that when I look to You, I find hope, I find help, and I find courage and strength. Help me to live each day in the light of Your glory and grace. Amen.

—— DAY 7: REFLECTION AND APPLICATION

Lord Jesus, You are the author of my faith, the finisher, the perfector; You are the pioneer, the champion, the victor. I'm running with my eyes fixed on You.

Write this week's memory verse:

_____

_____

Race Notes & Grace Notes

Where have you found grace for the race this week? Where did you make progress or take positive steps in the right direction?

_____
_____
_____

Where did you struggle or stumble? What obstacles did you face?

_____
_____
_____

What have you learned that you want to take with you, going forward?

_____
_____
_____

What do you want to let go of or leave behind?

_____
_____
_____

What other glimpses of grace —grace upon grace— has God given you this week?

_____
_____
_____

"Take the very hardest thing in your life—the place of difficulty, outward or inward,
and expect God to triumph gloriously in that very spot.
Just there, He can bring your soul into blossom."
—Lilias Trotter

Thank You, God, that nothing is beyond Your ability to redeem and restore. I'm holding tight to the hope that gives me. With every step I'm surrounded, strengthened, and sustained by Your mercy and grace.

End Notes

1. Janet Holm McHenry, Training For Success (Galveston: First Place for Health, 2015), 13.

2. Pam Farrel, Becoming a Brave New Woman: Step Into God's Adventure for You (Eugene OR: Harvest House Publishers, 2009), 218.

3. Kendra Smiley, Mother of the Year: 365 Days of Encouragement for Devoted Moms (Savage MN: Broadstreet Publishing, 2017), January 10.

4. Lauraine Snelling, Facebook post, April 11, 2023.

5. Jane Rubietta, Resting Place: A Personal Guide to Spiritual Retreats (Westmont IL: InterVarsity Press, 2005), 191.

6. Asheritah Ciuciu, Full: Food, Jesus, and the Battle for Satisfaction (Chicago IL: Moody Publishers, 2017), 100-101.

7. Lilias Trotter, "Focused: A Story & a Song." https://www.unveiling.org/lily/focussed.html.

Note: Lilias Trotter and Helen Lemmel were contemporaries who inspired each other. When Trotter heard the song Lemmel had written based on her devotional pamphlet, she republished it to include Lemmel's lyrics.

8. Helen Lemmel. 1922. "Turn Your Eyes Upon Jesus." Public Domain.

WEEK FOUR: GRACE TO LET GO

SCRIPTURE MEMORY VERSE

Commit everything you do to the Lord. Trust Him, and he will help you. **Psalm 37:5**

Some of us are trying to run this race with our shoelaces untied—or worse, tied together! And we can't understand why we just keep falling down. It seems we've been holding on to some really unhealthy mindsets that trip us up again and again in every area of our lives.

Maybe we're trying to move toward a healthier body, healthier marriage, healthier friendships, healthier finances, or healthier career or ministry. Whatever our goal is, here are five of the biggest hazards—the most dangerous attitudes—guaranteed to wreak havoc on our race:

1. I can't do this. I'm just going to fail (or fail again).
2. I want to do it perfectly or not at all.
3. I won't rest until I get it right.
4. I should be where they are. My race should look like theirs and so should my results.
5. I want those results to come easily and be obvious and instant.

Any of these mindsets resonate with you?

Every one of them has tripped me up at some point in my race—sometimes all of them at once! Holding on to them has held me back for far too long, especially because so much of what I'm trying to hold onto is beyond my control.

I find I constantly need to remember the wise words of author and Bible teacher Barb Roose, who writes: "There will always be circumstances out of our control, and the only path to God's power, peace, and provision in the midst of those circumstances is to surrender. Letting go and living like Jesus will sustain us, strengthen us, and set us up to experience God's best and beautiful blessings, not only in this life but also in the life to come."[1]

How do we let go and live like Jesus? The Bible tells us Jesus trusted His Father. He committed everything to Him and focused daily on walking in obedience to His Father's will. We can do this too, one step at a time.

That's our challenge this week. We're going to look at what God says about each of the mindsets that trip us up and ask Him to help us let go of them, surrender, trust Him, and commit ourselves and our race to Him.

—— DAY 1: TRY, TRY AGAIN

Lord Jesus, please be my Leader, my Teacher, my Trainer this week. Daily transform my heart and mind with Your Truth.

It's not easy to let go of our fears and step out in faith, to try to accomplish something that can feel so daunting—so impossibly hard—especially if we've tried and failed before. But we can do this. And we will. We are not doomed or destined to fail (or fail again). We have the best Coach in the universe behind us, before us, and beside us. The Scripture reminds us that with God nothing is impossible. All things are possible with Him (Matthew 19:26).

Let's look at what else God's Word tells us:

Read Isaiah 43:16-19. Who is the Lord? What "impossible" thing has He done before?

_____

_____

_____

What does He say He will do?

_____

_____

_____

Where do you need Him to be your Way Maker today?

_____

_____

_____

Now turn to Isaiah 35:1-4. What is the encouraging, good news?

_____

_____

_____

How do these verses speak specifically to you?

_____

_____

_____

Take a look at Philippians 3:10-14. What were Paul's goals?

_____

_____

_____

What was his attitude?

_____

_____

_____

How do Paul's words inspire you?

_____

_____

_____

There is freedom waiting for you,
On the breezes of the sky,
And you ask "What if I fall?"
Oh but my darling, What if you fly?[2]
—Erin Hanson

_____

_____

_____

God, thank You for being the wind beneath my wings, the strength and the power that enable me to soar above every obstacle, every fear and doubt. I know You will make a way for me today. Amen.

—— DAY 2: AIM FOR PROGRESS, NOT PERFECTION

Father, my heart's desire is to bring glory and honor to You. Help me to do that today, one choice at a time, one step at a time, one day at a time.

In Matthew 5:48 Jesus said, "Be perfect, even as your Heavenly Father is perfect." Be perfect? Well, it couldn't be impossible, if He said to do it, could it? So what did He mean?

If we do a little word study and dive deeper into this verse, we learn that the word often translated in English as perfect actually means "complete, whole, fully-developed." Not error-free. Not mistake-free. Not sinless—at least not in this life. Instead, we are on our way to being who God created us to be.

The Amplified Bible translates Matthew 5:48 this way: "Be perfect [growing into spiritual maturity both in mind and character, actively integrating godly values into your daily life], as your heavenly Father is perfect."

Sounds a little more do-able, doesn't it? This is good, because no matter how hard we try, we can't run this race without ever making any mistakes. When it comes to our health and wellness, we can't eat perfectly, track perfectly, and exercise perfectly every single day from now on, starting today (or Monday or next month or after the holidays). We have to let go of that idea.

It's hard, especially for those of us who are perfectionists by nature. But if we get stuck in all-or-nothing thinking—if we refuse to show ourselves the grace God has given us and throw in the towel every time we mess up, even a little bit, we'll never get anywhere. It's true of everything in life. I know you've heard it before, but that's why our goal is progress, not perfection (at least, not perfection in the usual sense of the word).

In Galatians 3:3 Paul reminds us that the only way we run this race at all is through the power of the Holy Spirit; we can never become perfect (grow strong, healthy, mature, and complete) by our own human effort. It's only by God's grace and in His strength.

So, we just do what we can do today. We keep making small changes, small choices, small steps in the right direction, even when we've just taken what feels like a huge step back. Especially then!

What does James 1:2-4 say about not giving in easily, not giving up when the going gets tough? Why should we persevere?

_____

_____

_____

What does 2 Corinthians 4:1 say?

_____

_____

_____

What does Galatians 6:9 promise?

_____

_____

_____

What do Lamentations 3:22-23 and Psalm 42:8 remind us?

_____

_____

_____

I love how The Message describes the kind of resilience God calls us to in Colossians 1:9-12:

> Be assured that from the first day we heard of you, we haven't stopped praying for you, asking God to give you wise minds and spirits attuned to his will, and so acquire a thorough understanding of the ways in which God works. We pray that you'll live well for the Master, making him proud of you as you work hard in His orchard. As you learn more and more how God works, you will learn how to do your work. We pray that you'll have the strength to stick it out over the long haul—not the grim strength of gritting your teeth but the glory-strength God gives. It is strength that endures the unendurable and spills over into joy, thanking the Father who makes us strong enough to take part in everything bright and beautiful that he has for us.

How do these truths speak to your life—your race—today?

_____

_____

_____

Lord, I'm asking You to deliver me from all-or-nothing thinking today. Help me to recover quickly when I make a mistake and be satisfied with doing my best for You. Give me Your strength. Show me how to lean in to Your mercy and grace.

—— DAY 3: WALK AWAY

Father, You know how easy it is for me to become obsessed—and then distressed—with how I perceive my performance. Help me to let go and look to You instead.

Yes, this race is important. Yes, we need to give it our best. Yes, God calls us to press on and persevere. But not without rest. Not without grace or mercy or forgiveness. Not in a spirit of desperate striving, driving ourselves, even punishing ourselves at a pace we can never maintain.

Look up Isaiah 40:11. How does God lead His people?

_____

_____

_____

What does Jesus offer us in Matthew 11:28-30?

_____

_____

_____

In Colossians 3:12-13, we're told how God wants us to treat others—it's the way He Himself treats us. Read these verses from this perspective, not as a to-do list for you, but as a description of God's heart toward you. What do you see?

_____

_____

_____

How does this match up with your perception? How does it match up with your own self-talk?

_____

_____

_____

If this is an area of struggle for you, take a few moments to listen to Andrew Peterson's song "Be Kind to Yourself" (look it up on YouTube or your favorite music streaming service).

It's easy to be unkind to ourselves, to be impatient and unloving and unforgiving—to push so hard that we wear ourselves out and cause significant harm or lasting damage. It's happened to me. There was a time when I got so fixated on the number on the scale, so frustrated and desperate and determined to see it change, that I did things I knew were unhealthy—even dangerous. For some months I deliberately mimicked some of the behaviors of people I knew who battled disordered eating. I'm thankful for a moment I will never forget — a moment when the Holy Spirit convicted me that if I didn't stop immediately, I would be enslaved to this disordered eating for real. That day, I called three trusted friends and confessed to them what I had been doing. I asked them to hold me accountable on a daily basis by asking me very specific questions I would have to answer honestly and specifically until those behaviors no longer had a hold on me. It was hard and humbling (honestly, humiliating), but I did it, and—thank God—I found freedom. (If I hadn't, I would have gone on to the next step: to seek professional counseling or treatment or whatever it took, as God showed me.)

If you find yourself in this place or close to it, you may find more help in My Place for Discovery, in the Be Free study, and in the book Truly Fed: Freedom from Compulsive Eating and Dieting by First Place for Health author Gari Meacham. You may also want to consider talking to a Christian counselor with experience in this area. As Beth Moore says, "I may walk with a spiritual limp, but thanks be to God, who holds me up and urges me to lean on Him, at least I can walk. So can you. Walk away from that pit before it's the death of you."[3]

To be kind to yourself and obedient to Jesus, what do you need to walk away from today?

_____

_____

_____

Where do you need help or support or accountability? How will you find it? What steps will you take?

_____

_____

_____

Lord, thank You for being so kind and loving and tender and patient with me. Thank You for giving me life and hope and healing and victory. Amen.

—— DAY 4: YOU DO YOU

Jesus, today I'm keeping my eyes on You and running the race You have called me to. Help me not to be distracted by other runners and their results. I just want to do my best for You.

How fast and how far and how long this race takes you is determined by a lot of factors. First and foremost are God's plans and purposes for you, the ones He established before the foundation of the world, the ones He had in mind when you were just a twinkle in His eye. (See Jeremiah 29:11 and Psalm 139.)

Your race won't look the same as others — even if they're in the same race, headed for the same finish line. You have different strengths, weaknesses, personalities, backgrounds, and experiences. You face different physical, mental, emotional, and spiritual challenges. You may be at different ages and stages of life or at different stages of the race itself. Comparing yourself and your results to them and theirs doesn't get you anywhere.

Put Galatians 6:4-5 in your own words.

_____

_____

_____

The Message paraphrases it this way:

> *Make a careful exploration of who you are and the work you have been given, and then sink yourself into that. Don't be impressed with yourself. Don't compare yourself with others. Each of you must take responsibility for doing the creative best you can with your own life.*

How (or when or where or with whom) are you most tempted to compare yourself? How do you feel when you do?

_____

_____

_____

What does it look like for you to "do the creative best you can with your own life"?

_____

_____

_____

What does Galatians 5:25-26 advise us?

_____

_____

_____

What does Proverbs 14:30 warn?

_____

_____

_____

What wisdom do you find in Romans 12:10-18 and Hebrews 10:24 that you can apply to your relationships with other runners in the race of faith?

_____

_____

_____

In light of the verses we've read, what will you choose to let go of today? What will you hold on to? What specific action will you take?

_____

_____

_____

God, help me today to support, encourage, and celebrate others—not envy them, compare myself to them, or compete with them in unhealthy ways. My race is my own, and following You, I will find victory.

—— DAY 5: KEEP IT REAL

Lord, don't let me get lost in fantasy scenarios. Help me to be honest about where I am and how I got here. When I think about what I can do and what it takes to grow and change, help me to keep it real.

The magazines at the grocery store checkout promise to teach me the secret to losing forty-three pounds in two weeks. *I really wish I could get those kinds of results! I should at least be able to lose ten or twelve pounds in two weeks, like I did that one time on that crash diet in my early twenties.* I go to the gym three times a week for three weeks, and I don't see any muscles forming. I'm telling you; I ate healthy every day this week. Oh wait, I forgot about Thursday. Okay it was probably more like five out of seven days. Or four. Hey, I ate healthier . . .

So why do my goals still feel so far out of reach?

Even on those rare days and weeks, when I really do pull it together and do everything right—at least everything I can possibly do—there are all kinds of forces at work, factors that I can't control.

I'm disappointed when I expect—even demand—obvious and immediate results. If there's one thing that both science and the Bible teach us, it's that growth takes time. Change takes time. Progress takes time. Wholeness and healing take time. Maturity (or "perfection") takes time.

My friend Jennifer Dukes Lee has written an entire book about it—*Growing Slow*—that, much as I love her, I did not want to read because I want things to be quick and easy. I think most of us do. But that's not how this works. It's not how God works.

Lee writes, "Sometimes the day-to-day growth is imperceptible, but I have to believe it's happening. I have to believe God designed us to develop spiritual maturity and obedience over time. It seems to me that God is interested in incremental growth as we develop habits of obedience, deep trust, and holiness . . . learning over time, through struggles, and in the midst of disappointment what it truly means to trust Jesus."[4]

It's true as we learn to trust Him with every part of our race, our journey — physically, mentally, emotionally, and spiritually.

Read each of the following passages and record what you learn about God's timing:

Ecclesiastes 3:1-11	
Isaiah 30:18	
Habakkuk 2:3	
Romans 8:24-28	
Romans 15:4	
2 Peter 3:8-9	

As Maggie Wallem Rowe reminds us, "We can wait anxiously and impatiently, or we can wait hopefully and expectantly, knowing God has not forgotten us. His arms are not too short to reach into our present situation. His silence does not equal His absence . . . God is at work in the wait."[5]

Thank You, God, for growing me slow—being patient with me, making time for me, and taking the time it takes. I know that one day I will rejoice in all that You have been working in and through me.

—— DAY 6: REFLECTION AND APPLICATION
Lord, You've searched me and You know me. You know my anxious thoughts. Calm my troubled heart and keep me in Your perfect peace today.

Years ago, I remember attending a women's conference. I was smiling on the outside, but on the inside, I was falling apart. Everything in my life was spinning wildly out of control. I'd been working hard to hold it together, but I just couldn't do it. So many of the things that were weighing on me were beyond my power to control.

There was nothing I could do—at least nothing I could see in my own wisdom, in my own strength. But that hadn't kept me from trying. Now here I was, frustrated, upset, anxious, worried, and worn out from all the fruitless effort.

Jennifer Kennedy Dean took the platform and told a story about a time when she went to an outdoor market with one of her young sons. Someone gave him a big helium balloon tied to a string. Jennifer warned her little boy more than once to hold on tight. But sure, enough the next time she turned around, he was searching the sky for a last glimpse of his precious balloon. Anticipating tears or a tantrum, she scolded him, "Honey, I told you to hold on tight! Why did you let go?"

Her toddler replied, "I didn't let it go, Mommy! I gave it to Jesus."

Jennifer's story made me cry, because—well, what a sweetheart! And because his answer is also for you and for me.

There are so many things in this life we just can't control. The answer is "let it go," but the only way we can let it go is if we're giving it to Jesus because we really don't want to walk away from the things and people who are important to us. We can't just abandon our responsibilities and commitments or our health and wellness goals. We don't want to ignore them or give up on them.

We don't just let these things go: we entrust them to the Creator of All Things. We give them to the One who is so much stronger, so much wiser, so much more just, good, patient, loving, and kind. He knows what to do so much better than we do. Sometimes when we step back and take a deep breath, He'll unfold a little of His plan and give us a task, something He wants us to pray or say or do. Other times He'll show us that He can take care of it all by Himself.

But either way, the difference it makes is huge! It's hard to describe the relief, the peace, the freedom. So when the temptation comes again—the temptation to try to control what you can't control, don't hold tight and don't just let it go. Give it to Him.[6]

Use the space on the following page to draw one big balloon or a bunch of balloons that you will label with the names of people or things you need to give to Jesus today. Place your hand over your drawing and pray a prayer of release. Picture the balloon(s) flying up to Him, and hold onto that image throughout the day.

Lord Jesus, I need Your help! Help me to let go of the things that are weighing on me. Please take all of these things that are too heavy for me and carry them for me. Please carry me today. Amen.

—— DAY 7: REFLECTION AND APPLICATION

God, Help me to let go of anything and everything that keeps me from running this race for You. Help me to look to You, trust You, and commit everything I do to You.

Write his week's memory verse:

_____

_____

_____

Race Notes & Grace Notes

Where have you found grace for the race this week? Where did you make progress or take positive steps in the right direction?

_____

_____

_____

Where did you struggle or stumble? What obstacles did you face?

_____

_____

_____

What have you learned that you want to take with you, going forward?

_____

_____

_____

What do you want to let go of or leave behind?

_____

_____

_____

What other glimpses of grace —grace upon grace— has God given you this week?

_____

_____

_____

"No matter what happens in my life, I live as a person of faith who knows how the story ends—God wins. And when my life on earth is finished, I rest in the assurance that I will see Jesus face to face. I also live each day in the way I want to be remembered, and trust that my own story and legacy has made a difference in someone's life. And for the kingdom."
—Lucinda Secrest McDowell

Lord Jesus, thank You for the overwhelming victory You have promised me. Thank You for the work You are doing—even now—in and through me. Thank You for the grace that carries me. Thank You for the love that sustains me. Amen.

End Notes

1. Barb Roose, Surrendered: Letting Go and Living Like Jesus (Nashville: Abingdon Press, 2020), 12.

2. Erin Hanson, Reverie: The Poetic Underground #1 (Morrisville NC: Lulu, 2014), 57.

3. Beth Moore, Get Out of That Pit: Straight Talk about God's Deliverance (Nashville: Thomas Nelson, 2017), 88.

4. Jennifer Dukes Lee, Growing Slow: Lessons on Un-hurrying Your Heart from an Accidental Farm Girl (Grand Rapids: Zondervan, 2021), 32.

5. Maggie Wallem Rowe, This Life We Share: 52 Reflections on Journeying Well With God and Others (Colorado Springs: NavPress, 2020), 76.

6. Christin Ditchfield, What Women Should Know About Letting It Go: Breaking Free from the Power of Guilt, Discouragement, and Defeat (Abilene TX: Leafwood Publishers, 2015), 139-140.

5 Dietrich Bonhoeffer, The Cost of Discipleship (New York: Simon and Schuster, 2012), 45.

6 John Wesley, The United Methodist Hymnal (Nashville: Abingdon Press, 1989), Number 607.

WEEK FIVE: GRACE TO LEARN AND GROW

SCRIPTURE MEMORY VERSE

So take a new grip with your tired hands and strengthen your weak knees. Mark out a straight path for your feet so that those who are weak and lame will not fall but become strong. **Hebrews 12:12-13**

I bet if I played you the first three seconds of the Academy Award-winning theme, you'd picture the film scene immediately: a group of Olympic athletes in the 1920s, running through the chilly waves on a foggy British beach.

Like every great sports movie or superhero movie or movie about someone discovering (or reclaiming) who they were meant to be, Chariots of Fire features epic training montages. As viewers we follow the protagonists through a series of clips that show them in some kind of training program, struggling and stumbling, learning and growing. Often the characters are shown broken down and exhausted by the process, but then they persevere until they're built back up again, confident, focused, and energized.

The background music from these movies makes a great workout playlist—one I often use to motivate me as I train for a big race. But on my toughest days, it's actually a sermon that inspires me—again, from Chariots of Fire.

In my head I hear Olympian and missionary Eric Liddell preaching to a crowd gathered round him:

You came to see a race today. To see someone win. It happened to be me. But I want you to do more than just watch a race. I want you to take part in it. I want to compare faith to running in a race. It's hard. It requires concentration of will, energy of soul . . . I have no formula for winning the race. Everyone runs in her own way, or his own way.

Then he asks this question: "Where does the power come from, to see the race to its end? From within. Jesus said, 'Behold, the Kingdom of God is within you. If with all your hearts, you truly seek Me, you shall ever surely find Me.' If you commit your-self to the love of Christ, then that is how you run a straight race."[1]

After that, I hear the actor who plays Liddell, quoting from Isaiah 40:28-31 (KJV) in a voiceover, as we see the other runners competing for Olympic glory:

Hast thou not known? hast thou not heard, that the everlasting God, the Lord the Creator of the ends of the earth, fainteth not, neither is weary? . . .

He giveth power to the faint; and to them that have no might He increaseth strength . . .

But they that wait upon the Lord shall renew their strength; they shall mount up with wings as eagles; they shall run, and not be weary; and they shall walk, and not faint.

This week we're talking about the moments that would make up our own training montage—how we learn from victory and from defeat and how we tap into the strength that carries us when we're weak and weary, the strength that comes from within.

—— DAY 1: LEARN FROM VICTORY

Lord, I thank You for each and every victory You've given me and for what You are teaching me today as I run this race.

Read Psalm 18:1-6, 16-19, 30-39. (You may want to underline key words or phrases that resonate with you.) How did the psalmist find victory? How was he prepared to achieve this?

What did victory look like?

What else do you learn from these verses?

_____

_____

_____

Turn to Psalm 40:1-3. What did victory look like in this scenario and what brought it about?

_____

_____

_____

How did the psalmist respond to this victory? What did he expect would be the result?

_____

_____

_____

Not every victory is obviously epic. Not every battle is won on a stage big enough for all the world to see. But as author Deb Gruelle points out, "We create a legacy for those who come after when we take small faithful steps that align with our values each day. Each choice to follow God (or not) matters. We offer what we have to Him. It's up to God to do the miracles."[2] And He does. Faithfully and consistently.

What steps have you taken—big or small—that have led to victory? What strategies have you learned that work for you?

Physically:

_____

_____

_____

Mentally:

_____

_____

_____

Emotionally:

_____

_____

_____

Spiritually:

_____

_____

_____

Take a few moments to celebrate these things and thank God for the things He's taught you:

_____

_____

_____

By God's grace and in His strength, how can you build on these victories?

_____

_____

_____

God, You are my strength and my victory. All the glory and honor and praise belong to You.

—— DAY 2: LEARN FROM DEFEAT

God, thank You for using everything, even my struggles and stumbles, my failures and defeats, for my good—my growth—and Your glory.

Twice I have been swept from the course (picked up by race staff in a shuttle) while attempting a half marathon. Once I was swept at ten miles because I had just not disciplined myself to train properly or consistently in the months leading up to the race. The second time I got eight miles in, but again I wasn't strong enough or fit enough and I was in too much pain—though I'm also going to blame that one on an unexpected surgery three months earlier that derailed my training.

Both times I was walking on my own. I hadn't been able to convince any of my friends or family to join me. I didn't have any support or accountability—either for the training or for the race. I wonder if I might have found the strength to finish if I'd had good company. (We'll talk more about this on Day 3.)

Over the years I think I've learned as much from my defeats as I have from my victories. I've learned what types of exercise I don't enjoy or can't fit easily into my schedule. I've learned what nutritional approaches don't work for me and my body. I've learned when I'm most vulnerable to temptation and what triggers me to over-eat. I've learned how to bounce back and get back on track as many times as it takes in a given week. Lately I've learned that I can't count on having the resolve to start over tomorrow or Monday. The best thing I can do is focus right now on the choice I have right in front of me.

What about you? What has not been working for you?

Physically:

_____

_____

_____

Mentally:

_____

_____

_____

Emotionally:

_____

_____

_____

Spiritually:

_____

_____

_____

Clinical educator and nutrition researcher Megan Ramos says, "It's never failure and always a lesson."[3] Others have put it this way: "It's not failure, it's feedback"—infor-mation that you can use to finetune things.

So what have you learned? What can you do differently?

Physically:

_____

_____

_____

Mentally:

_____

_____

_____

Emotionally:

_____

_____

_____

Spiritually:

_____

_____

_____

Jesus never failed, but the Bible tells us He did learn from His suffering. What did He learn, according to Hebrews 5:8?

_____

_____

_____

Look up Philippians 4:10-13. What did Paul learn from his suffering?

_____

_____

_____

What else did he learn, as recorded in 2 Corinthians 1:8-10?

_____

_____

_____

According to 1 Corinthians 2:1-4, what did Paul learn from his experience ministry? (For background, see Acts 17:16-34.)

_____

_____

_____

Poet Maya Angelou famously said, "Do the best you can until you know better. Then when you know better, do better."

In Psalm 119:7, the psalmist exclaimed, "As I learn Your righteous regulations, I will thank You by living as I should!"

Use these words to help you form a prayer of your own that you can pray this week:

_____

_____

_____

Thank You, God, for turning my defeats into victories, to the glory of Your name.

—— DAY 3: LEARN FROM EACH OTHER

Lord Jesus, thank You for the people You have called to come alongside me, those I can learn from and who are a source of inspiration, comfort, and strength.

Yesterday I mentioned how much harder it was for me to run a race alone when I didn't have anyone to encourage me, support me, or push me to dig deep and persevere. In My Place for Fitness, Mary Ward reminds us, "Studies show that those who exercise with a friend or group find more success and accountability. And asking a friend to join you might just be the motivation your friend needs to get moving!"[4]

That's why, whenever I can, I recruit friends and family to race with me because it's good for them and it's good for me! The Scripture tells us that "iron sharpens iron" (Proverbs 27:17) or as we often say in First Place, "we are better together." We take turns supporting and encouraging one another, challenging one another, and cheering for one another. When one wins, we all win!

It's true not only when it comes to our health and wellness, but also in every other part of life with every kind of race we run.

What did Paul urge believers to do in 1 Thessalonians 5:11 and Hebrews 10:24?

_____

_____

_____

What does Paul urge us in Philippians 2:4 and Romans 15:1?

_____

_____

_____

As The Message paraphrases this week's memory verse, Hebrews 12:12-13:

Don't sit around on your hands! No more dragging your feet! Clear the path for long-distance runners so no one will trip and fall, so no one will step in a hole and sprain an ankle. Help each other out. And run for it!

That kind of help can make all the difference in the world.

When I signed up for my very first half marathon, I asked my little sister to join me. On race day at mile 10, we found ourselves climbing a steep on-ramp up to the highway. At that point I was already exhausted and in a lot of pain. In between gasps for air, I told Stephanie I was scared, I was getting dizzy, and I felt I might actually fall backward if I couldn't get some momentum going—it was that steep.

Without saying a word, she dropped behind me, balled up her fist, and pushed it firmly into my lower back—as if to steady me and propel me forward—and she kept it there, all the rest of the way up the ramp.

I will never forget how much that helped me mentally and emotionally and even spiritually, much more than it did physically. I get teary thinking about it even now. It's become a powerful image for me of God's grace in giving us faithful companions to run this race with us—the fist in our back or the "wind beneath our wings."

So who runs this race with you? And who is in your cheering section? Whom do you turn to when you need support, encouragement, or accountability? (There may be different people who play different roles and provide help in different ways.)

Whom do you run with or for? And whose cheering section are you in? Whom do you support, encourage, or hold accountable? (There may be different people that you are called to help in different ways.)

_____

_____

_____

Who can you strengthen and support today or this week? Specifically, what will you do?

_____

_____

_____

Lord Jesus, thank You for the people You have called to come alongside, those I can support and encourage and teach and those I can be an example and an inspiration to. Help me to faithfully point them to You.

—— DAY 4: LEARN FROM YOUR WEAKNESS

Father, help me to be as patient with myself as You are with me, and to rest in the love that You have for me.

Earlier this week, we talked about learning from our defeats. The reality is that we will all experience both victory and defeat—sometimes on the same day, sometimes in the same hour, or even in the same minute. We all have good days and bad days. We have strengths and we have weaknesses. It's how we were made.

Author, speaker, and life coach Georgia Shaffer reminds us, "Accepting the good and bad in ourselves isn't easy, but it is essential if we are going to heal and be free to move on. So let go and give Jesus your pain and disappointment. Don't be weighed down by condemnation. Reject any voices in your head that are continually reminding you of your wrongs. Remember the truth of Romans 8:1: '. . . there is now no condemnation for those who are in Christ Jesus.'"[5]

What did Paul say in 2 Corinthians 12:8-10 when he was confronted with his own weakness? What did he learn?

_____

_____

_____

What was his attitude, going forward?

_____

_____

_____

Look up each of the following verses and record what you learn about our weakness and God's heart toward us:

Psalm 103:13-14	
Isaiah 53:4-5	
Matthew 12:20	
Romans 8:26	
1 Corinthians 15:43	
Hebrews 4:15	

What promise do we find in 1 Corinthians 1:8?

_____

_____

_____

How do these verses speak to you? How can they shape your attitude toward God and yourself and the race you are running today?

_____

_____

_____

Thank You, Jesus, for being so gentle with me, so patient and understanding. Thank You for Your mercy and grace. Thank You for Your strength at work in and through me. Thank You for the hope of glory.

—— DAY 5: LEAN ON HIS STRENGTH

God, You are the Source of my strength, my courage, my wisdom, my peace. You have given me all of these things to help me run my race because You love me and You want me to succeed.

The Message paraphrases 1 Corinthians 1:8-10 this way:

Just think—you don't need a thing; you've got it all! All God's gifts are right in front of you as you wait expectantly for our Master Jesus to arrive on the scene for the Finale. And not only that, but God Himself is right alongside to keep you steady and on track until things are all wrapped up by Jesus. God, who got you started in this spiritual adventure, shares with us the life of his Son and our Master Jesus. He will never give up on you. Never forget that.

In *Unafraid* author and speaker Gracie Malone says, "All of us live a grace story. God does not accept us or love us because we're special, because we deserve to be loved, or because we are attractive or brilliant (or unattractive and a bit dense). He loves us because of grace. Before we even believe in Him, He draws us to Himself by grace. We choose to believe because His grace enables us to see the truth and accept it. We experience a lifetime of graceful interventions as we follow His plan for us. And the best part? Grace helps us today, right where we are, enabling us and giving us the power to do what we cannot do ourselves."[6]

How did God's people become victorious, according to Psalm 44:3?

_____

_____

_____

Turn to Hebrews 12:14-17 and 1 Peter 2:1-3. What can trip us up and keep us from experiencing God's grace and strength?

_____

_____

_____

Remember that in Genesis 25:27-34, Esau let his physical hunger drive him to agree to a terrible bargain with his brother Jacob. Esau gave up his birthright and all the special blessings he was to inherit in the future —for a bowl of stew.

The writer of Hebrews exhorts us to "Watch out for the Esau syndrome: trading away God's lifelong gift in order to satisfy a short-term appetite. You well know how Esau later regretted that impulsive act and wanted God's blessing—but by then it was too late, tears or no tears" (Hebrews 12:17 MSG).

What should we desire more than the immediate gratification of our physical needs? (See 1 Peter 2:2-3)

_____

_____

_____

What do Proverbs 4:23 and 2 Timothy 1:13-14 urge us to do for our own wellbeing?

_____

_____

_____

What does Paul pray that God will do in 2 Thessalonians 2:16-17?

_____

_____

_____

What does God promise in Isaiah 41:10?

_____

_____

_____

How can the truths we've talked about here help you to lean on God's strength to help you run your race today?

_____

_____

_____

End your time today with this prayer by Jennie Afman Dimkoff:

"Dear Heavenly Father, thank You for encouraging me. Please forgive me for the times I've wallowed in my circumstances rather than keeping my eyes on You and following Your direction. Please breathe Your wisdom into me and let it be apparent in my speech and in my actions. Help me to honor You with my life and to be open to Your leading. Father, I struggle with old hurts. Please give me Your capacity to forgive, because I simply can't in my own strength. And Father, please drain the pain from those old wounds and heal me from the inside out! Help me to focus on the future that You have for me, instead of the past. Thank You for loving me and for the plan You desire to work out in my life. In the precious Name of Jesus, Amen."[7]

—— DAY 6: REFLECTION AND APPLICATION

God, thank You for Your grace, thank You for Your truth, thank You for Your light. Give me eyes to see the beauty in running this race You've called me to, and the beauty in this world You have made.

We've been talking a lot about running this race of faith—running, training, battling, fighting, persevering, pressing on, overcoming. Somewhere in there, there also needs to be some resting.

And not just resting in the sense of trusting—like resting on God's promises or resting in His love for us—but resting in His presence. Being still, not striving. Resting from our labors, even the good work He's given us to do. Resting our hearts, our minds, our spirits, and our bodies.

Even in the middle of our training, we need time for rest and recovery. In Rhythms of Rest, Shelly Miller talks about how God Himself has built rhythms or seasons of rest into Creation.

"On the sixth day, God didn't say, 'I'm finished' — full stop — as a justification for a day of rest on the seventh. God is in the business of continually creating, and His work is never fully finished. The work you have to do while you are on this earth is never fully finished either. Sabbath isn't an allowance for when the dishes are done, projects are complete, or when your volunteerism is on hiatus... Sabbath is the exhale required after six days of inhaling our work."[8]

Do you hear what she's saying? Rest isn't something you earn. It's a commandment you obey. And like all of His commandments, it's a gift from God to you—meant to provide for you and protect you.

Remember Eric Lidell? He was really big on Sabbath-keeping, honoring God by setting aside regular time for worship and prayer and rest. He was willing to sacrifice his Olympic dreams if they threatened to keep him from doing so.

How are you doing with Sabbath-keeping? Do you build in time to rest on a regular basis? If not, how could you?

_____

_____

_____

Sundays stopped being a day of rest at our house when my husband became a pastor—but we try to take at least one day a week to honor the spirit of Sabbath. As Shelly says, "Jesus is Sabbath. [However we do it] when we make the day different on His behalf, holiness inhabits our intentions."[9]

_____

_____

_____

What does rest look like to you? What refreshes and renews you? What recharges or re-energizes you?

Physically:

_____

_____

_____

Mentally:

_____

_____

_____

Emotionally:

_____

_____

_____

Spiritually:

_____

_____

_____

Don't be legalistic about it (that's missing the point entirely, just like the Pharisees). But see how many of these practices you can incorporate into your schedule on a regular, ongoing basis.

Remember the promise of Jesus, who said, "Come to Me, all who are weary and heavily burdened [by religious rituals that provide no peace], and I will give you rest [refreshing your souls with salvation] (Matthew 11:28 AMP).

Thank You, Lord, for the rest You promise me. Help me to make room in my life to receive it today.

—— DAY 7: REFLECTION AND APPLICATION

Father, the depth of Your love and Your mercy and Your grace amazes me. I'm so grateful for Who You are and for what You do, in and through me.

Write this week's memory verse:

_____

_____

_____

Race Notes & Grace Notes
Where have you found grace for the race this week? Where did you make progress or take positive steps in the right direction?

_____

_____

_____

Where did you struggle or stumble? What obstacles did you face?

_____

_____

_____

What have you learned what you want to take with you, going forward?

_____

_____

_____

What do you want to let go of or leave behind?

_____

_____

_____

What other glimpses of grace —grace upon grace— has God given you this week?

_____

_____

_____

"Jesus comes not for the super spiritual but for the wobbly and the weak-kneed who know they don't have it all together, and who are not too proud to accept the handout of amazing grace."
—Brennan Manning

Thank You, Lord, for the gift of Your grace. Jesus, I know how desperately I need it! My heart and my hands are open to receive all that You have for me today. Amen.

End Notes

1. Chariots of Fire, directed by Hugh Hudson (Hollywood: Warner Bros. Pictures, 1981). Note: On YouTube, you can watch brief clips of the scenes quoted in the introduction.

2. Deb Gruelle, "From a Small Act of Obedience," Small Steps Blog, May 4, 2017, https://debgruelle.com/small-steps-blog/fromasmallactofobedience/.

3. Megan Ramos, The Essential Guide to Intermittent Fasting for Women (Vancouver, Canada: Greystone Books, 2023), 243.

4. Mary Ward, My Place for Fitness (Galveston TX: First Place for Health, 2018), 67.

5. Georgia Shaffer, "Help! I Can't Forgive Myself! How To Finally Let Go of Regret to Find Ultimate Freedom" Georgia Shaffer Blog, September 30, 2022, https://georgiashaffer.com/uncategorized/stories/i-cant-forgive-myself/.

6. Gracie Malone, Unafraid: 365 Days Without Fear (Brentwood TN: FaithWords, 2015), 328.

7. Jennie Afman Dimkoff, Passionate Faith: Ancient Truths for Contemporary Women (Grand Rapids: Our Daily Bread, 2015), 118-119.

8. Shelly Miller, Rhythms of Rest: Finding the Spirit of Sabbath in a Busy World (Bloomington MN: Bethany House, 2016), 16-19.

9. Shelly Miller, Rhythms of Rest, 19.

WEEK SIX: GRACE TO BELIEVE

SCRIPTURE MEMORY VERSE
No discipline is enjoyable while it is happening—it's painful! But afterward there will be a peaceful harvest of right living for those who are trained in this way. **Hebrews 12:11**

It takes a lot of courage and determination and self-discipline to run this race. And sometimes we just don't have it—or enough of it. Sometimes we get distracted and wander off track. Or we get turned around somehow and run in the wrong direction.

Sometimes—like a certain eight-year-old I once did a Fun Run with—we have a bad attitude. We grumble and whine and complain with every step we take (which I'm telling you right now is not fun for anyone).

Sometimes we convince ourselves we're doing our best—giving it our all—but we really aren't. Sometimes we're being stubborn or rebellious or just really good at making excuses.

Thankfully, as we talked about in Week 3, we have the World's Best Coach and Personal Trainer (who also happens to be our Heavenly Father). And He won't let us get away with anything. Not if it's going to harm us or others—or cause harm to our relationship with Him. Not if it's going to keep us from running this race victoriously—crossing the finish line and receiving our trophy.

The Scripture tells us He loves us enough to discipline us—to teach us, train us, and yes, to correct us. He loves us enough to tell us when we've gotten off track and to help us make the appropriate course correction. He loves us enough to get our attention when we're distracted or making careless mistakes (and He'll use whatever it takes). He'll challenge us to grow up and get over our bad attitudes because the race is hard enough to run without a massive chip on our shoulder. And He'll motivate us to dig deep, deeper than we thought possible. That's where we'll find strength we didn't know that we could have and do things we never dreamed we could do.

No, it's never fun to be disciplined or corrected. It can be painful in the moment. But it's super helpful in the long run. (Pun intended.)

Notice that as we talk about this important truth this week, we're going to steer clear of the word punishment—even if that's a word that some of our Bible translations use—because it can have a lot of baggage. In the world we live in, punishment is not always deserved. It's not always just or fair. It's not always constructive—intended for the good (for the benefit) of the one being punished. We often use the word punitive to describe something harsh, cruel, and unforgiving. And that's not the character of our Heavenly Father at all.

Sometimes we punish ourselves or our bodies out of guilt and shame in an effort to make ourselves pay for or in some way make up for (atone) for our sins. And that's bad theology. Jesus has already atoned for our sins. He paid the penalty in full. He still lovingly corrects us, disciplines us, teaches us, and trains us, but only in a truly redemptive way. Only for our good.

Let's talk more about this.

—— DAY 1: BELIEVE IN HIS GOODNESS

Lord, teach me to trust You completely—trust in Your goodness, Your mercy, Your grace. Open my heart to hear what You're saying to me today.

Let's look more closely at the context of this week's memory verse. Read Hebrews 12:1-11. This is a familiar chapter and we've already explored the first few verses in detail. But this time we're paying particular attention to verses 5-11. Notice that in verse 5 the writer of Hebrews refers to the words in verses 5 and 6 (taken from Proverbs 3:11-12) as encouraging words—which might not be how we would first be inclined to describe them.

So why does God discipline us—and how is this supposed to be encouraging? (See verses 6-8, 10.)

How should we respond to discipline and correction? (See verses 5, 7, 9.)

How is God's discipline different from other discipline we may have received? What promises do we find in Hebrews 12:10-11?

_____

_____

_____

Here's how The Message paraphrases this passage. As you read it, underline key words and phrases that resonate with you.

Have you forgotten how good parents treat children, and that God regards you as His children?

> My dear child, don't shrug off God's discipline,
> but don't be crushed by it either.
> It's the child He loves that He disciplines;
> the child He embraces, He also corrects.

God is educating you; that's why you must never drop out. He's treating you as dear children. This trouble you're in isn't punishment; it's training, the normal experience of children. Only irresponsible parents leave children to fend for themselves. Would you prefer an irresponsible God? We respect our own parents for training and not spoiling us, so why not embrace God's training so we can truly live? While we were children, our parents did what seemed best to them. But God is doing what is best for us, training us to live God's holy best. At the time, discipline isn't much fun. It always feels like it's going against the grain. Later, of course, it pays off big-time, for it's the well-trained who find themselves mature in their relationship with God.

In *Fresh Hope for Today*, Grace Fox reminds us,

> You and I are running a long-distance race . . . If we hope to endure and finish well, we must lay aside those things that hinder us. Unbelief is a common hindrance that affects our progress. Doubting God's goodness, wisdom, and power paralyzes us. The good news is that the heroes of the faith shed unbelief and ran their race by faith in God's promises. They endured and finished strong, and we can do the same.[1]

Take a few moments to listen to Chris Tomlin's song "Good Good Father" and/or CeCe Winans' "Goodness of God" (you can find them on YouTube or your favorite music streaming service). Or choose another favorite praise and worship song.

Write an affirmation or prayer declaring what you believe about who God is and why you can trust Him and His discipline today.

_____

_____

_____

Father, Thank You for Your love for me, thank You for Your faithfulness to me, thank You for working in and through me today. Amen.

—— DAY 2: BELIEVE IN THE PROCESS

God, I believe that You have my best interests at heart, and that everything You do is for my good and Your glory. I love You, and I trust You with my life today.

Look up Psalm 103:8-14. How does this Psalm describe God? (See verses 8, 13.)

_____

_____

_____

Is this how you were raised to think of God? Is this how you think of Him now?

_____

_____

_____

How does God discipline us, according to this psalm? What does He do? What does He not do? (See verses 9-10, 12.)

_____

_____

_____

Why does He do and not do these things? (See verses 8, 11, 14.)

_____

_____

_____

How have you experienced God's discipline in the past or how are you experiencing it now?

_____

_____

_____

Have you resisted or responded? (Or are you now resisting or responding?) In what ways?

_____

_____

_____

What have you learned or are you learning?

_____

_____

_____

King Hezekiah experienced a life-threatening illness that he described as God's discipline. What did he testify in Isaiah 38:15-17?

_____

_____

_____

What declaration of faith does the psalmist make in Psalm 71:20-21?

_____

_____

Thank You, God, that You are willing to do whatever it takes to teach me and train me and that You do it so lovingly, so tenderly, so patiently. Thank You for the good things Your discipline will produce in me and all the blessings You have in store for me.

—— DAY 3: BELIEVE IN PAIN'S PURPOSE

Lord, I believe that any kind of pain or suffering You allow in my life—regardless of its source—is an opportunity. It serves a greater purpose when it points me to You.

From beginning to end, the Bible promises us that our "good, good Father" is sovereign—that nothing happens that is not part of His perfect will (what He orchestrates and causes to take place) or His permissive will (what He doesn't cause, but allows). Everything we experience—including our weakness and our failures and mistakes—serves His greater purpose for us.

Let's look at what we learn about the purpose of God's discipline and correction in Isaiah 30:15-26.

What did God's people need to learn? (See verses 15-17.)

_____

_____

_____

What do we need to learn about God? (See verses 18-19.)

_____

_____

_____

What does God promise in verses 19-21, Proverbs 4:11-12, and Psalm 32:8?

_____

_____

_____

What is our part in all of this? What action do we take? (See Isaiah 30:15, 19.) How should we respond to what God is teaching us? (See verse 22.)

_____

_____

_____

What would be the result, according to verses 23 and 26)?

_____

_____

_____

How can you relate what we've read today to your health and wellness journey?

_____

_____

_____

Christian author and fitness professional Alisa Keeton reminds us,

No challenging moment surprises God. He has signed off on every moment of your life, and each is designed to help conform you more into the image of Christ. Let's be people who trust God with our pain, who go to Him to stay loose and shake off our stress, rather

than people who stay rigid and blame God for our adversity. We will encounter troubles, but we can be quick to metabolize our pain by going to God. This is how we prevent pain from having the last word and make it useful for God's glory. Adversity comes with a gift, the potential for us to have greater intimacy with God and become more Christ-like.[2]

What kind of pain are you experiencing in your life right now and how is God using it? What purpose is it serving?

_____

_____

_____

Holy Spirit, show me how to make the most of this pain—how to receive it as a gift and allow it to do its work. Give me the patience, courage, and strength to endure it, in Jesus' name.

—— DAY 4: BELIEVE IN THE SACRIFICE

Lord Jesus, You sacrificed everything for me: You endured the pain and the shame of being crucified on the cross. Help me be willing to sacrifice—willing to endure pain and hardship—for Your sake.

In her book *Don't Quit, Get Fit* First Place for Health national director Vicki Heath quotes "The Competitor's Creed" recited by the Fellowship of Christian Athletes. Vicki points out how appropriate it is for all of us running this race of faith—and the race to greater health and wellness. It reads in part:

> *My body is the temple of Jesus Christ.*
> *I protect it from within and without.*
> *Nothing enters my body that*
> *does not honor the Living God.*
> *My sweat is an offering to my Master.*
> *My soreness is a sacrifice to my Savior.*
>
> *I give my all—all of the time.*
> *I do not give up. I do not give in.*
> *I do not give out. I am the Lord's warrior—*
> *a competitor by conviction*
> *and a disciple of determination.*

> *I am confident beyond reason*
> *because my confidence lies in Christ.*
> *The results of my efforts*
> *must result in His glory.[3]*

Heath writes,

Just let those words sink in for a minute. This is the ultimate motivation we have been looking for. This describes making our sacrifice out of love and devotion to the Savior. At the end of my boot-camp classes, we huddle up, say this prayer and then wipe our brows and hold out our sweat offerings for the Lord. We make the sacrifice and then we pray that God will find our offerings acceptable and pleasing.[4]

Vicki is referencing Romans 12:1-2. The Message paraphrases the passage this way:

So here's what I want you to do, God helping you: Take your everyday, ordinary l i f e — your sleeping, eating, going-to-work, and walking-around life—and place it before God as an offering. Embracing what God does for you is the best thing you can do for Him . . . Fix your attention on God. You'll be changed from the inside out. Readily recognize what He wants from you, and quickly respond to it. Unlike the culture around you, always dragging you down to its level of immaturity, God brings the best out of you, develops well-formed maturity in you.

How might this perspective be a game-changer for you?

_____

_____

_____

In *Everything Is Yours* my dear friend Kris Camealy talks about a time she felt God calling her to sign up to run a race to raise money for a Christian children's charity. Answering this call would be much harder than going online and making a donation. To keep her commitment to God and to the charity, she would have to get serious about her health and wellness. She would have to go into training, changing her eating habits and prioritizing her exercise routine. She would have to make time for this in the midst of her already super-busy life. It would require sacrifice.

Kris found it was an intense battle—every bit as much mentally, emotionally, and spiritually, as it was physically. She had to stop making excuses, stop listening to her own negative self-talk, and ignore phantom pains, distractions, and discouragements. Surrender has been a big theme in her spiritual life, and looking back, she writes,

This time, surrender didn't look like being still, or resting in God's presence. This time, surrender had been a hard-scrabble push to do something that was beyond my own strength. In this, God taught me that sometimes surrender looks more like pressing into what feels impossible, and learning to trust that God is both able and willing to carry us when we step out into the hard places of obedience.[5]

Where is God calling you to obedience?

_____

_____

_____

What is He asking you to sacrifice or surrender as part of your training?

_____

_____

_____

In Psalm 51 King David is responding to God's discipline and correction. In verse 17 what kind of sacrifice does he say God wants?

_____

_____

_____

What kind of sacrifice does Psalm 141:2 describe?

_____

_____

_____

What kind of sacrifice does Hebrews 13:15 call us to make?

_____

_____

_____

How can making these daily sacrifices help you run your race?

_____

_____

_____

God, I know that everything I am and everything I have is Yours—a gift from You, a gift I'm giving back to You with love and gratitude today.

—— DAY 5: BELIEVE IN THE OUTCOME

Jesus, Your discipline and correction and redirection are exactly what I need. I believe You have good things in store for me.

All week, we've been touching on the rewards that come when we choose to respond to God's discipline with obedience, sacrifice, and surrender. Flip back through Days 1-4, and see if you can list some of these positive outcomes— the fruits, the harvest, the results:

First Place for Health author Karen Porter reminds us,

God not only dwells in us, He delights in us. He does not leave us drifting without purpose. He sees the great in our future. Even when we think we are doing well, He has bigger plans. God's agenda is to set us free from the bonds of self and the attitudes and mindsets poured in by family and experiences. His plans are greater, bigger, and higher than any strategy or scheme we've mapped out. He isn't interested in what we think we can be. He is interested in transforming every part of us, because God intends to make us like Christ. The question is, will I cling to little modifications, or will I allow total change? Will I embrace what He has arranged?[6]

How would you answer those questions?

Look up the following verses from Psalm 107 and fill out the chart below, identifying the crisis, how those in crisis responded to their plight, and the result or outcome:

Psalm 107	Crisis	Response	Outcome
1-9			
10-16			
17-20			
25-30			

What else does God do for His people, according to Psalm 107:33-38?

_____

_____

_____

What does Psalm 107:43 tell us?

_____

_____

_____

Over the course of our lives, there will be many times when we need God's discipline, correction, and training—lovingly given to us for the purpose of bringing us to a new place of wisdom, strength, growth and maturity.

And sometimes He orchestrates a radical course correction or redirection. Author Jill Swanson asks,

Have you ever felt like God was [completely] restyling or repurposing your life? I think we experience this kind of process every time we encounter a major change—such as the beginning or end of a relationship, career, or ministry, a pregnancy, a job promotion or job loss, a serious or chronic illness, retirement, empty nest . . . the list goes on and on. When we see that a particular season is coming to an end, we can feel like our purpose and usefulness is ending, too—when in reality, God is getting us ready for what's next. He's preparing us for the next adventure, a new beginning. If you have a pulse, you have a purpose—and God has a plan![7]

How would you describe the race you're running today? After being off track, is God calling you to get back on track or just run with more focus and intention in the same direction, or is He leading you in a new or different direction?

How do you feel about it? If you are seeking a different outcome, what's the hardest thing for you to change?

It isn't always easy to persevere when we don't know God's plan, when we don't see any fruit or harvest yet, or when the race seems unending. But as author Cynthia Ruchti says, "God speaks to a listening heart, and one of His messages during those 'I can't do this anymore' days is '[I know. I'm here.] My power is made perfect in your weakness' (see 2 Corinthians 12:9 NIV)."[8]

Thank You, Father, that I can do all things through Christ who strengthens me. I can trust You for the outcome, because You keep Your promises and fulfill Your plans and purposes for me. Show me the next step You want me to take. "Speak, Lord, for Your servant is listening."

—— DAY 6: REFLECTION AND APPLICATION

God, give me the grace to persevere through difficult seasons and the grace to trust that You will make a way through.

Sometimes we find ourselves in what seems like an impossible situation—caught between the armies of Pharaoh and the Red Sea (see Exodus 14). We face all kinds of obstacles that complicate our best efforts to "run with perseverance the race marked out for us" (Hebrews 12:1 NIV).

The worst part is that sometimes we have a part in the problem. With our health and wellness, for instance, we may be dealing with the result of decades of poor choices, bad habits, a lack of discipline or self-control, and half-hearted attempts to change. We may be in dire straits. It can be really daunting.

But nothing is impossible with God. And He isn't finished with us yet. He hasn't given up on us. The situation isn't hopeless as it seems.

In *The Red Sea Rules* Robert J. Morgan reminds us,

> *The blood of Jesus Christ forgives our sins and resolves our guilt. His resurrection frees us from the fear of death, and it satisfies our need for eternal significance and happiness. The presence of the Lord surrounds us, while the promises of the Bible sustain us. His grace heals our whip wounds. Jesus said, "Therefore if the Son makes you free, you shall be free indeed" (John 8:36).*

But Satan doesn't surrender his prey without a fight. He comes racing after . . . chariot wheels churning the dust, seeking to discourage you, to defeat you . . .

He tries to trap you in difficulty, to entangle you in trouble, to corner you in impossible situations, to lure you into temptation. If you're in a tough situation right now, suffering pain, worry, anguish, or illness, the devil is undoubtedly behind it to a greater or lesser degree.

Acknowledge Satan's activity, but don't be intimidated by him. You can resist him in the power of God, by the blood of Jesus Christ . . .

When we rebuff the enemy in the name of Jesus Christ, when we stand our ground, when we resist his wiles and claim the victory of faith, when we shake off discouragement in the name of our Lord, Satan falls from heaven faster than lightning. He is drowned in the Red Sea of the blood of Jesus Christ.[9]

Hallelujah! Like the children of Israel, we will praise God from the opposite shore: "I will sing to the Lord, for He has triumphed gloriously; he has hurled both horse and rider into the sea. The Lord is my strength and my song; he has given me victory" (Exodus 15:1-2).

Use the space below to list as many things as you can think of that have been swept into the sea, drowned, washed away, or covered by the blood of Jesus today.

_____

_____

_____

_____

_____

_____

_____

_____

Thank You, Jesus, for Your blood that was shed for me. Thank You for the victory You have already won. Thank You for forgiveness and fresh mercies.

—— DAY 7: REFLECTION AND APPLICATION

Lord Jesus, thank You for loving me exactly as I am—but too much to leave me this way. Thank You for teaching me, testing me, training me, and transforming me by Your grace.

Write this week's memory verse:

_____

_____

_____

Race Notes & Grace Notes
Where have you found grace for the race this week? Where did you make progress or take positive steps in the right direction?

_____

_____

_____

Where did you struggle or stumble? What obstacles did you face?

_____

_____

_____

What have you learned that you want to take with you, going forward?

_____

_____

_____

What do you want to let go of or leave behind?

_____

_____

_____

What other glimpses of grace —grace upon grace— has God given you this week?

_____

_____

_____

"The meaning of life. The wasted years of life. The poor choices of life.
God answers the mess of life with one word: 'grace.'"
—Max Lucado

Lord Jesus, thank You for the hope You give me each and every day. Thank You for the help and strength You give me. Thank You for the grace.

End Notes

1. Grace Fox, Fresh Hope for Today: Devotions for Joy on the Journey (Peabody MA: Aspire Press, 2022), 115.

2. Alisa Keeton, The Body Revelation (Carol Stream IL: Tyndale, 2023), 76.

3. "The Competitor's Creed," The Fellowship of Christian Athletes, https://www.fca.org/resources/the-competitor's-creed/read-the-competitor's-creed.

4. Vicki Heath, Don't Quit, Get Fit: Overcoming the 4 Fitness Killers (Ventura CA: Regal, 2011), 92.

5. Kris Camealy, Everything Is Yours: How Giving God Your Whole Heart Changes Your Whole Life (Westerville OH: Refine Media, 2019), 71.

6. Karen Porter, If You Give a Girl a Giant: Fighting for Your Life (Friendswood TX: Bold Vision Books, 2019), 37.

7. Jill Swanson with Christin Ditchfield, 30 Day Makeover Inside and Out (Friendswood TX: Bold Vision Books, 2021), 140.

8. Cynthia Ruchti, As My Parents Age: Reflections on Life, Love, and Change (Franklin TN: Worthy, 2017), 270.

9. Robert J. Morgan, The Red Sea Rules: 10 God-Given Strategies for Difficult Times (Nashville: Thomas Nelson, 2014), 34-35.

WEEK SEVEN: GRACE TO RECEIVE

SCRIPTURE MEMORY VERSE

The temptations in your life are no different from what others experience. And God is faithful. He will not allow the temptation to be more than you can stand. When you are tempted, He will show you a way out so that you can endure.
1 Corinthians 10:13

There will always be a reason not to run your race today—a reason you "can't" make wise, healthy, God-honoring choices. A reason you don't have the time or energy. A reason to treat yourself. A reason to take a break from your training program. A reason to call it a day, with the promise to get back on track tomorrow.

Sometimes it's a good reason—a reasonable reason. Totally legit. Sometimes it's an excuse, a rationalization, a form of procrastination.

Sometimes it's a temptation.

The dictionary defines temptation as a strong desire to do something that is wrong or unwise. It's an urge or an impulse to act in a way that goes against your best interests.

Biblically speaking, temptation is a test or a challenge but also an opportunity to exercise discipline and self-control, to do the right thing (instead of the wrong thing), to walk in faithfulness and obedience to God. Or not.

The Bible tells us that God doesn't tempt us: "Remember, when you are being tempted, do not say, 'God is tempting me.' God is never tempted to do wrong, and he never tempts anyone else" (James 1:13).

Theologian Thomas Aquinas described temptation as coming from three different sources: "the world, the flesh, and the devil."[1] This week we're going to look at how each of these sources conspires against us and how we can overcome them.

It's important to know that experiencing temptation isn't a sin. We all experience temptation—even Jesus was tempted by Satan in the wilderness (Matthew 4:1-11). It's when we give in that the sin comes in.

God allows us to be tempted because it's an opportunity to win a victory—to become strong in the mighty power of God. The alternative is to struggle, stumble, learn a thing or two, and receive the grace that will help us recover and enable us to resist the temptation (or at least resist longer) in the future.

All you need to remember is that God will never let you down; He'll never let you be tempted past your limit. He'll always be there to help you come through it (1 Corinthians 10:13 MSG).

—— DAY 1: THE WORLD

God, be my Strength and my Shield today. Give me victory over temptation, I pray, in Jesus's mighty Name.

Let's think about the temptation we experience that comes from the outside world—anything external to us that is opposed to the Kingdom of God as well as anything that would distract us, discourage us, or defeat us as we seek to live a life worthy of our calling and run with perseverance the race marked out for us.

Circle below the worldly sources of temptation that you are most conscious of, and add specific examples — or any other sources that come to mind:

- Advertising—on TV and websites, on billboards, in magazines and apps, or on social media with seasonal or special sales

  _____

  _____

- Peer pressure—from family and friends, coworkers, neighbors, and other influencers

  _____

  _____

- Society in general and social situations—holiday celebrations, office parties, church picnics and potlucks, girls' or guys' nights out

  _____

  _____

- Other:

  _____

  _____

What does 1 John 2:15-16 warn us?

_____

_____

_____

What does 1 Corinthians 7:23 remind us?

_____

_____

_____

What does 1 Peter 2:11 urge us?

_____

_____

_____

According to 2 Peter 1:3-10, what has God given us? What will all this do for us?

_____

_____

_____

How should we respond? (See verses 5-10.)

_____

_____

_____

Why should we respond this way (vs 8, 10-11)?

_____

_____

_____

How can you apply these truths to your battles with temptation and the race you're running today?

_____

_____

_____

We will brainstorm some more specific strategies for resisting temptation on Day 5. If you want to, you can go ahead and do that exercise with a worldly temptation you've identified today.

Father, thank You for all that You have promised me—including victory over tempta-tion! Help me to love You and listen to You and follow You—not the way of the world—today.

—— DAY 2: THE FLESH

Lord, lead me not into temptation. My spirit is willing, but my flesh is weak. Forgive me. Have mercy on me, and make haste to help me.

In 2023 the number one song at the top of the Billboard charts for weeks on end was performed by a young woman reflecting on how she had repeatedly refused to learn from her mistakes, how she avoided taking responsibility for her own self-sabotaging behavior — to her own heartache, grief and shame. In the chorus, she finally con-fessed that she herself was the problem.[2]

There's a reason the lyrics resonated with so many people. Sometimes we are the problem—we can be our own worst enemy.

What does James 1:14-15 tell us about this source of temptation?

_____

_____

_____

How did Paul describe this problem in Romans 7:14-24?

_____

_____

_____

Can you relate? Where do you experience this in your own life?

_____

_____

_____

In *When You Pray* Philip Graham Ryken observes,

The weaknesses we see in the people of the Bible are the very weaknesses we ought to rec-ognize in ourselves. Like Eve, who ate the forbidden fruit, we are vulnerable to temptation when we act on our own. Like Abraham, who lied about his wife to save his neck, we are vulnerable to temptation when we are scared. Like David, who slept with Bathsheba while his men were off to war, we are vulnerable to temptation when we are idle. Like Elijah, who wanted God to end his life, we are vulnerable to temptation when we are exhausted. Like Peter, who denied his Lord even after he promised to die for him, we are vulnerable to temptation when we are overconfident. In other words, we are vulnerable to temptation practically all the time.[3]

According to Paul in Romans 7:25 and 8:1-2, what is the hope—what is the answer?

(Again, we'll look at forming specific strategies for facing specific temptations that we find ourselves vulnerable to in the exercise on Day 5.)

Martin Luther is quoted as saying, "God delights in our temptations and yet hates them. He delights in them when they drive us to prayer. He hates them when they drive us to despair."[4]

How does 2 Corinthians 7:10 explain this?

What does Acts 3:19-20 urge us to do? Why? What will happen next?

Take a few moments to quiet your heart. Ask the Holy Spirit to show you anything you need to confess and repent of, and write your prayer in the space below:

You might also use these words from The Book of Common Prayer:

Most merciful God, we confess that we have sinned against you in thought, word, and deed, by what we have done, and by what we have left undone. We have not loved you with our whole heart; we have not loved our neighbors as ourselves. We are truly sorry and we humbly repent. For the sake of your Son Jesus Christ, have mercy on us and forgive us; that we may delight in Your will, and walk in your ways, to the glory of your Name. Amen.[5]

—— DAY 3: THE DEVIL

Lord, if You are for me, who can stand against me? Step by step, day by day, You lead me to victory, for the glory of Your name.

You know, I've never participated in a 5k, 10k, or half marathon in which the spectators were rooting against me (they just aren't like that!). I've never had another runner purposely trip me or bump into me or injure me. Running (or walking) is an individual sport—there's no opposing team, no enemy. But in the race of faith, it's a different story.

You and I have a wicked enemy who will stop at nothing to ruin everything.

He tries to keep us from signing up and tries to keep us from ever starting the race to begin with. And when that doesn't work, he tries to distract us, get in our heads, and play mind games. He tries to fill us with fear and doubt and tries to discourage us. He boos us and threatens us. He throws all kinds of dangerous obstacles in our path—anything to confuse us, injure us, slow us down, or knock us off track. And if he can't make us quit, he'll do his best to make us miserable. He's pretty mad that we escaped his clutches in the first place.

Ephesians 2:2 says, "You used to live in sin, just like the rest of the world, obeying the devil—the commander of the powers in the unseen world. He is the spirit at work in the hearts of those who refuse to obey God."

Look up Colossians 1:13-14 and Colossians 2:13-15. What changed for us? How did we escape?

According to John 10:10, what does the enemy — "the thief"—want? What have we been given that he wants to take from us?

_____

_____

_____

What does 1 John 4:4 remind us?

_____

_____

_____

How does 1 Peter 5:8-9 describe this enemy?

_____

_____

_____

How should we respond to his attacks? Why?

_____

_____

_____

Turn to the story of Jesus' temptation in Luke 4:1-13. Why do we need to continue to stay alert (see verse 13)?

_____

_____

_____

According to Romans 8:37, what's the good news that we can cling to today?

_____

_____

_____

Lord Jesus, deliver me from evil and from the evil one today. Help me to stand firm, stay strong, and fight hard with all the wisdom, courage, and strength that You give me. Thank You for the victory You have promised me.

—— DAY 4: THE PRAYER

Father, help me to call on You when I'm in over my head—and even when I think I've got this. Especially then. I desperately need Your grace, moment by moment, day after day.

C.S. Lewis was once making an argument against the idea that "bad people" really can't help themselves, because they suffer so much temptation—it's just so hard for them—and that "good people" are only good because (for whatever reason) they really aren't tempted to do wrong—they just don't know how hard it is, because "they don't know what temptation means."

Lewis wrote,

> *Only those who try to resist temptation know how strong it is . . . A man who gives in to temptation after five minutes simply does not know what it would have been like an hour later. That is why bad people, in one sense, know very little about badness. They have lived a sheltered life by always giving in.*

Now that's a different perspective, isn't it? The truth is that resistance is hard! But it is never futile. The Bible reminds us to look to Jesus—and keep looking to Him always—especially in the heat of the battle.

As Lewis says,

> *We never find out the strength of the evil impulse inside us until we try to fight it: and Christ, because He was the only Man who never yielded to temptation, is also the only Man who knows to the full what temptation means.*[6]

What does Hebrews 4:15 tell us about His attitude toward us and our battles?

_____

_____

_____

Hebrews 12:4 reminds us that we have not yet struggled as much and fought as "agonizingly against sin, nor have you yet resisted and withstood to the point of pouring out your [own] blood" (AMPC).

When did Jesus do this? Look up Luke 22:39-44.

What did He tell His disciples to pray?

What did He pray?

How and when could you pray this prayer in your life today?

Write it in your own words.

Yes, Lord, I'm saying "no" to temptation and "yes" to You today. Yes to Your will, yes to Your way, yes to Your tender mercy and amazing grace.

—— DAY 5: THE PLAN

Lord Jesus, You know all about temptation—wherever it comes from—and how to resist it. Teach me Your ways. Give me a heart of wisdom and the will to obey.

Think of a specific temptation that has troubled you and prayerfully answer each of the following questions. (You may remember them from your school days—the 5 Ws and an H):

WHO is tempting me?

_____

_____

WHAT am I being tempted with?

_____

_____

WHEN am I being tempted?

_____

_____

WHERE am I being tempted?

_____

_____

HOW (specifically) am I being tempted?

_____

_____

WHY am I being tempted? (What need do I have that this temptation promises to meet?)

_____

_____

Now let's use a variation of these questions to help us find a successful strategy for dealing with this temptation—a "way of escape" (1 Corinthians 10:13).

WHOM can I turn to for help or support when I face this temptation? (And how will I do that?)

_____

_____

WHAT do I want more than this temptation is offering me?

_____

_____

WHEN will I take action and prepare to battle this temptation?

_____

_____

WHERE can I flee? How can I avoid this situation altogether—or get out of it quickly?

_____

_____

If I can't flee, HOW can I resist? How can I address the underlying need that's driving me in a God-honoring way?

_____

_____

WHY do I want to resist this temptation? Why is it worth fighting? What might my reward be?

_____

_____

Note that you can use this exercise in any area in which you experience temptation— in any part of your race, not just your health and wellness journey.

As Hebrews 4:16 reads in The Amplified Bible:

Therefore let us [with privilege] approach the throne of grace [that is, the throne of God's gracious favor] with confidence and without fear, so that we may receive mercy [for our failures] and find [His amazing] grace to help in time of need [an appropriate blessing, coming just at the right moment].

Thank You, God, that You've got me and I've got You. I know I can go the distance because Your grace is enough for me. I receive that grace, that mercy, that strength wholeheartedly. I thank You and I praise You, in Jesus's name. Amen.

—— DAY 6: REFLECTION AND APPLICATION
Lord Jesus, You know all about temptation—wherever it comes from and how to resist it. Teach me Your ways. Give me a heart of wisdom and the will to obey.

I mentioned spectators earlier this week. Even the most casual, low-key races have them—folks who get up ridiculously early and brave the cold (or the wind or the heat), put on funny hats or face paint, grab their pom-poms and cowbells and root for their friends and family—perhaps like the "cloud of witnesses" in Hebrews 12. The cool thing is that as long as they're standing there on the sidelines, these spectators will cheer for everybody! Even if they don't know you, they'll offer you a thumbs up or a high five. Some hand out bottled water. Many of them hold up homemade signs. These signs may have a simple message: "You can do it!" or just a runner's name. Some have pictures of the runner or a picture of the person in whose honor or in whose memory they're running. Others feature dad jokes, clever puns, or movie quotes.

I can tell you from experience that reading all these signs really helps pass the time. It keeps the miles flying by. A good sign can distract you from the pain of your sore muscles, make you grin or giggle a little, or touch your heart. It can encourage and inspire you, remind you of your purpose, and assure you that it's all going to be worth it when you cross the finish line. It's true, even when the sign wasn't made with you in mind. I think my favorite was "I'm so proud of you, random stranger!"

Today I'm inviting you to make your own sign—using a verse we read this week, a catchphrase, movie quote, or motivational saying. It could be a variation of "Keep Calm and ...." or a reminder of your "why." Something that will help you stay strong when you're battling temptation this week:

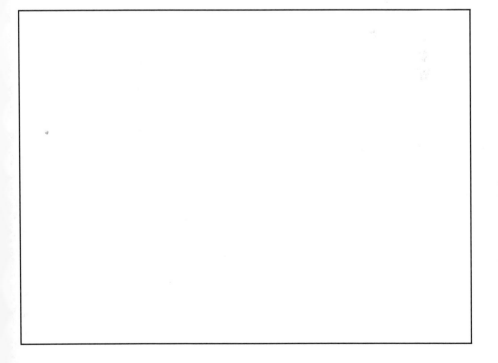

Why did you choose this message? What does it mean to you? What do you want to remember when you see it?

Now make a copy of your sign and paste it in your journal or stick it to your bathroom mirror. Or take a picture and use it as your home screen. Share it on social media or send it in a text message to someone you know who needs to hear the same thing.

Jesus, thank You for rooting for me! Thank You for cheering me on to victory. Thank You for the people in my life who come alongside me and support me. Thank You for the people I get to support, too.

—— DAY 7: REFLECTION AND APPLICATION

God, keep my eyes on You. Help me to find the way that You have made for me today. Help me to follow wholeheartedly after You.

Write this week's memory verse:

Race Notes & Grace Notes

Where have you found grace for the race this week? Where did you make progress or take positive steps in the right direction?

Where did you struggle or stumble? What obstacles did you face?

What have you learned that you want to take with you, going forward?

What do you want to let go of or leave behind?

_____

_____

_____

What other glimpses of grace —grace upon grace— has God given you this week?

_____

_____

_____

> "Remember that you're never alone in life and never without hope.
> Whether you're tempted, tired, or troubled, you can count on
> God's sustaining grace to uphold you."
> —Rick Warren

Yours, O Lord, is the battle, and Yours is the victory! Yours is the praise and the honor and the glory, now and forever. Amen.

End Notes

1. Thomas Aquinas, "Summa Theologica. Whether prudence of the flesh is a sin?" Christian Classics Ethereal Library (ccel). https://www.ccel.org/ccel/aquinas/summa.SS_Q55_A1.html. Retrieved 5 September 2023.

2. Taylor Swift, "Anti-Hero," Midnights. Republic Records, October 24, 2022.

3. Philip Graham Ryken, When You Pray (Wheaton IL: Crossway Books, 2000), 148.

4. Martin Luther, "Table Talk." Christian Classics Ethereal Library (ccel). https://www.ccel.org/ccel/luther/tabletalk.v.ii.html. Retrieved 5 September 2023.

5. The Episcopal Church. The Book of Common Prayer and Administration of the Sacraments and Other Rites and Ceremonies of the Church : Together with the Psalter or Psalms of David According to the Use of the Episcopal Church.(New York: Seabury Press, 1979), 360.

6. C.S. Lewis, Mere Christianity (Revised and Expanded Edition) San Francisco: (Harper One, 2001), 140.

WEEK EIGHT: GRACE TO GO THE DISTANCE

SCRIPTURE MEMORY VERSE

The God of peace will soon crush Satan under your feet. May the grace of our Lord Jesus be with you. **Romans 16:20**

Every race I have ever entered has turned out to be an epic journey—a test of endurance—not only physically, but also mentally, emotionally, and spiritually (not unlike my experience in the race of faith)!

From the moment I've clicked "register," I've experienced all kinds of thoughts, feelings, and emotions: excitement and anticipation, determination and motivation, anxiety and fear, weariness and misery and boredom (with all that training), and yes, joy and courage and strength. All of it culminates on the big day—race day —which goes something like this:

Me, at the starting line: I'm so excited! I can't believe I'm here, I'm doing this! I can do this. It's gonna be so awesome. Look at all the other amazing people out here. I'm so proud of us! I could hug everyone right now. I'm getting teary . . . Okay, focus. It's time. On your mark, get set . . .

Mile 1: Oh dear God. What was I thinking? Every muscle in my body is tight and tense and sore. My lungs are on fire. I can't breathe. Oh, what is happening? This is excruciating. If it hurts this much now, I won't even make it two miles, let alone thirteen. This was a terrible mistake!

Miles 2-3: I'll just go as far as I can—I mean, I have to. The paramedics aren't around at this stage. I'll just keep going until I collapse, and they appear. In the meantime I'll try to think how I can explain what happened to all the people I told I was doing this race.

Miles 4-5: Wait . . . you know, now that I'm warmed up, I'm not that sore anymore. I can breathe. I actually feel pretty strong. It feels good to move. Why was I so panicked? What was I so worried about? I've trained for this. I've found my rhythm, my pace. I can do this!

Mile 6: Okay, I'll admit this has been a good, long, vigorous walk. But I'm tired now and I'm over it. Seriously, I'm ready to be done. (If I'd signed up for the 10k, I WOULD be done.) Auughh! I don't want to do this anymore—certainly not for seven more miles. I'm not even halfway.

Mile 7: More than halfway—I'm more than halfway. God, help me!

Miles 8-10: Wait, is this like a second wind? Really? I feel strong again and the miles are flying by. This is amazing! I'm mean, I'm not saying I want to do this EVERY day, but I can do it today. It's doable. Just keep putting one foot in front of the other.

Mile 11: This is miserable. I hate this. Why did I sign up for this race? I'm never doing this again.

Mile 12: My whole body is aching. My feet feel like they're bleeding—every step is like walking on broken glass. But I'm so close, I know I'm going to finish this. I can finish this, and I never, ever have to do it again. I WILL never do this again. Almost there. I'm almost there.

Mile 13: Wait, where's the finish line? We're done, right? Are you kidding me— it's all the way down there? How can one-tenth of a mile feel longer than the whole rest of the race?

Me, staggering across the finish line: Oh thank You, Jesus. Thank You, Jesus. I can't believe I did it! I did it! Hooray! I'm so proud of myself. Oh the relief, the joy, the exhaustion—it's all hitting me, all at once. Thank You, Jesus! I did it. I proved to myself that I could—and I never have to do it again. Thank You, Jesus.

Me, posting photos on social media: "Had an absolute blast! So much fun!" (Which is true because once the temporary pain has passed, what remains is the thrill of victory, the sense of accomplishment, and the memories of special moments along the way.)

Me, a few months later, surfing online late at night: Oh look! Another race . . . cool medal! Cute t-shirt! Where do I register?

It may sound silly, but I promise this is what happens every single time. And it serves as a great reminder to me in just about every other area of my life: there are going to be highs. There are going to be lows. There will be all kinds of twists and turns, obstacles, and challenges to face. There will be many times when I feel like I can't take another step—when it seems impossible—or when I'm just totally over it (whatever "it" is).

But it won't always be this way. It will get better. I can get through it. I can do incredibly hard things. I know this, because the Word of God says so and because by God's grace and in His strength, I already have.

I can press on and persevere. And I know you can, too.

—— DAY 1: LISTEN UP

Lord, thank You for giving me grace to go the distance. Show me what that grace looks like in my life—in my race—today.

In every race, there are moments when it feels miserable, impossible, hopeless, endless! We lose sight of what we're running for. It's really hard. And we're really tired. We don't want to do this anymore. It's in these moments we need to hold tighter than ever to the truth of God's Word.

Read Psalm 16:8, 11. According to these verses, of what can we be sure?

_____

_____

_____

What does the psalmist declare in Psalm 56:13?

_____

_____

_____

What promise can we claim in Psalm 65:11?

_____

_____

_____

What does James 1:12 remind us?

_____

_____

_____

What does Galatians 6:9 urge us to do—and not to do? Why?

_____

_____

_____

What encouragement do these verses give you as you run your race today?

_____

_____

_____

Jesus, help me to remember that I can do all things through You, because You strengthen me and sustain me. You have already won the victory.

—— DAY 2: TAKE HEART

God, walk with me today. Be my strength and my song. Help me to persevere and press on, for the love of You, trusting in Your never-ending grace and mercy.

Remember it's not just our own human weakness that we fight to overcome. What does Ephesians 6:12 warn us?

_____

_____

_____

Read Ephesians 6:10-18. How should we respond? What should we do?

_____

_____

_____

What advice does Ephesians 6:18 give us?

_____

_____

_____

One of the most effective ways we can fight back against the enemy of our souls is to spend less time thinking of our own pain, our own suffering, and our own struggles and spend more time looking for ways to help others.

Take a moment to look at the runners all around you (metaphorically speaking). Who else is struggling or stumbling in their race? Who else is coming under attack? Whom can you fight for, pray for, and support and encourage in some way?

_____

_____

_____

What action can you take on their behalf today?

_____

_____

_____

Now read Psalm 121. Ultimately, where does our help come from?

_____

_____

_____

List some of the promises you find in this psalm—promises you can cling to and share with others.

_____

_____

_____

In his book *A Long Obedience in the Same Direction* Eugene Peterson writes that with every step we take, every breath,

We know we are preserved by God, we know we are accompanied by God, we know we are ruled by God; and therefore no matter what doubts we endure or what accidents we experience, the Lord will preserve us from evil, He will keep our life. We know the truth of Luther's hymn:

And though this world, with devils filled
Should threaten to undo us,
We will not fear, for God hath willed
His truth to triumph through us.
The prince of darkness grim,
We tremble not for him;
His rage we can endure,
For lo! his doom is sure;
One little word shall fell him.[1]

Hallelujah! Praise God! As Romans 8:37 says, "we are more than conquerors" (NIV)—"overwhelming victory is ours through Christ who loved us" (NLT). So let's walk on!

Thank You, Jesus, for loving us so much. Thank You for fighting for us, protecting and defending us, leading us to victory. We thank You and we praise You today.

—— DAY 3: TRUST GOD

God, help me not to give up when the going gets tough, but to be an overcomer. Show me the way today.

Many of us have been trying to lose weight and get healthy, fit, and strong for a very long time. Over the years, we have found victory . . . and lost it . . . found it again . . . and lost it again. In each season of life—each leg of the race—we find ourselves running into obstacles. Some are familiar, even constant. Some are new and unexpected. As we follow the course, we encounter places where the road suddenly narrows, and we feel "hard pressed on every side" (2 Corinthians 4:8 NIV).

Think about it for a few minutes: what are the biggest obstacles that you're facing right now? What makes it most challenging for you to run your race? What's getting in the way?

Make a list in the blank space on the following page or draw a simple, winding road and add assorted boulders (big and small circles) with the names of those obstacles.

Author Carol Kent says it's important to remember that "when we are stuck between a rock and a hard place, we have not reached the end of the road." These obstacles can actually become opportunities that lead to "a transforming and liberating encounter with the only true Rock—God Himself."[2]

This is her testimony, she says. This has been her experience:

"Year after year, God continues to transform my hard places into grace places where I discover surprising gifts of faith, mercy, contentment, praise, blessing, freedom, laughter, and adventure—tailor-made for me with His tender loving care."[3]

Take a few moments to read 2 Corinthians 4:7-18. How do these verses speak to your heart? What encouragement do you find?

Now spend a few moments in prayer. Talk to God about the specific obstacles you're facing. Thank Him for them, and ask Him to transform them into opportunities, into blessings, into "grace places" in your life today.

Father, keep reminding me that every obstacle I face is an opportunity to look to You for fresh courage and grace and strength.

—— DAY 4: PRESS ON

God, I believe that You are working all things together for my good—even the hard things, the hard days. Help me to persevere and press on today.

Yesterday, you took time to name the obstacles that you're facing right now. Today, set a timer for three minutes and use the space below to list obstacles that—by God's grace—you have already overcome OR "hard things" that you manage to do all the time.

_____

_____

_____

_____

_____

How did you do it? How do you do it? What got (or gets) you through it?

_____

_____

Take a look at Paul's list in 2 Corinthians 11:23-29. What had he experienced and by God's grace overcome? Jot down some of the highlights.

_____

_____

_____

Paul insists he's not going for gold in the Martyr Olympics here (that's what we call it in my family, when some of us get carried away describing our suffering, one-upping each other with our tales of woe: "You think that's bad . . . "). It's not about who's suffered more or longer or harder. Paul's not feeling sorry for himself either. He's not grumbling or complaining, and he's not getting discouraged or defeated by all these things.

What is his attitude, according to 2 Corinthians 12:10?

_____

_____

_____

What does he say about all this in Philippians 4:12-13? What is his secret?

_____

_____

_____

Practically speaking, what does this look like? How could he do this? How can we? Go back a few verses to Philippians 4:6-7, and list what Paul says to do.

_____

_____

_____

In Philippians 4:8-9, what strategy does he give us? What will help us persevere and press on, day after day? What will bring us victory?

_____

_____

_____

How can you apply this to your own race today? What are your takeaways?

_____

_____

_____

Holy Spirit, keep bringing to my mind all You have done in and through me and all You have taught me on this journey. Help me use every strategy, every weapon You've given me today, for Your Kingdom and Your glory.

—— DAY 5: HAVE FAITH

God, give me the faith to believe You will see me through and that every step I take is worth taking because it brings me closer to You.

In Hebrews 10:23-25, we find "A Call to Persevere." Look up these verses and list the three parts of this call:

1. _____

2. _____

3. _____

Why should we respond to this call? (See verses 23b and 25b.)

_____

_____

_____

What does answering this call look like for you? Write your answer for each part of the call:

1. _____

2. _____

3. _____

Now read Titus 2:11-14. Again, we're called to persevere in our race of faith (and our health and wellness journey). What are we called to turn away from? What does that look like today for you personally?

_____

_____

_____

What (and whom) are we called to turn to or look forward to? What does that look like today for you personally?

_____

_____

_____

Why should we answer this call? (See verse 14.)

_____

_____

_____

What does 1 Peter 1:6-7 call us to do? Why? What's the point—the greater purpose?

How does this give you perspective, challenge you, or inspire you as you run your race?

Lord, I believe in You, I hope in You, I trust in You. I love You. Thank You for loving me so tenderly and faithfully. Thank You for never giving up on me.

──── DAY 6: REFLECTION AND APPLICATION

Lord, this race sometimes feels long and lonely, but I know I am never alone. You are with me every step of the way. And step by step, day by day, You give me grace. You renew my strength.

Imagine with me that you're out there (somewhere) running your race—your heart is pounding even harder than your feet. Your breathing is heavy. You're hot and sweaty. Your muscles are aching. It's really tough. You're keeping your head down, just trying to put one foot in front of the other and trying not to think too hard about how far you might still have to go. Suddenly, in your peripheral vision, you see another runner coming up alongside you. It's your brother in Christ, Paul (the one who had all that great advice earlier this week). He's already run his race, already crossed the finish line, but he's come back to keep you company on this difficult stretch.

He's come because he wants to remind you what this race is all about. He has some encouraging words for you: You can do this! You've got this! Because God's got this—and God's got you!

It's true . . .

"Now God has us where He wants us, with all the time in this world and the next to shower grace and kindness upon us in Christ Jesus. Saving is all His idea, and all His work. All we do is trust Him enough to let Him do it. It's God's gift from start to finish!" (Ephesians 2:7-8 MSG)

"By entering through faith into what God has always wanted to do for us—set us right with Him, make us fit for Him—we have it all together with God because of our Master Jesus. And that's not all: We throw open our doors to God and discover at the same moment that He has already thrown open his door to us. We find ourselves standing where we always hoped we might stand—out in the wide open spaces of God's grace and glory, standing tall and shouting our praise." (Romans 5:1-2 MSG)

"We're not keeping this quiet, not on your life. Just like the psalmist who wrote, 'I believed it, so I said it,' we say what we believe. And what we believe is that the One who raised up the Master Jesus will just as certainly raise us up with you, alive. Every detail works to your advantage and to God's glory: more and more grace, more and more people, more and more praise!" (2 Corinthians 4:13-15 MSG)

"So we're not giving up. How could we! Even though on the outside it often looks like things are falling apart on us, on the inside, where God is making new life, not a day goes by without his unfolding grace. These hard times are small potatoes compared to the coming good times, the lavish celebration prepared for us. There's far more here than meets the eye. The things we see now are here today, gone tomorrow. But the things we can't see now will last forever." (2 Corinthians 4:16-18 MSG)

"Because we know that this extraordinary day is just ahead, we pray for you all the time—pray that our God will make you fit for what He's called you to be, pray that he'll fill your good ideas and acts of faith with His own energy so that it all amounts to something. If your life honors the name of Jesus, he will honor you. Grace is behind and through all of this, our God giving himself freely, the Master, Jesus Christ, giving himself freely." (2 Thessalonians 1:11-12 MSG)

"Receive and experience the amazing grace of the Master, Jesus Christ, deep, deep within yourselves." (Philippians 4:23 MSG)

"God be with you. Grace be with you." (2 Timothy 4:22 MSG)

How do these words speak to your heart today? What hope or encouragement do you find? (You might want to go back and underline or circle key words and phrases.)

_____

_____

_____

How will you respond? What will you do? What is the next step for you?

God, You've got me and I've got You. I know I can go the distance because Your grace is enough for me. I receive it wholeheartedly. I thank You and I praise You, in Jesus's name. Amen.

—— DAY 7: REFLECTION AND APPLICATION

Lord Jesus, thank You for all the grace You have given me—the many ways You have blessed me as I run this race. Help me to go the distance. Help me to stay strong and finish well for Your kingdom and Your glory.

Write this week's memory verse:

Race Notes & Grace Notes

Where have you found "grace for the race" this week? Where did you make progress or take positive steps in the right direction?

Where did you struggle or stumble? What obstacles did you face?

What have you learned that you want to take with you, going forward?

What do you want to let go of or leave behind?

_____

_____

_____

What other glimpses of grace —grace upon grace— has God given you this week?

_____

_____

_____

"Run each day's race with all your might, so that at the end you will receive the victory wreath from God. Keep on running even when you have had a fall. The victory wreath is won by him who does not stay down, but always gets up again, grasps the banner of faith and keeps on running in the assurance that Jesus is Victor."
—Basilea Schlink

God, You have been so good to me. And I know the best is yet to be! You have promised me victory so I will run and keep on running until I cross the finish line and run into Your arms. I will hear You say, "Well done!" And I will rest in Your love for me. Amen.

End Notes

1. Eugene H. Peterson, A Long Obedience in the Same Direction (Westmont IL: InterVarsity Press, 1980), 41.
2. Carol Kent, Between a Rock and a Grace Place (Grand Rapids: Zondervan, 2010), 18.
3. Carol Kent, Between a Rock, 19.

WEEK NINE: A TIME TO CELEBRATE

This week you have the opportunity to create a short victory celebration testimony. Work through the following questions in your prayer journal, one on each day leading up to your group's celebration.

DAY ONE: List some of the benefits you have gained by allowing the Lord to transform your life through this First Place for Health session. Be mindful that He has been active in all four aspects of your being, so list benefits you have received in the physical, mental, emotional and spiritual realms.

DAY TWO: In what ways have you most significantly changed mentally? Have you seen a shift in the ways you think about yourself, food, your relationships, or God? How has Scripture memory been a part of these shifts?

DAY THREE: In what ways have you most significantly changed emotionally? Have you begun to identify how your feelings influence your relationship to food and exercise? What are you doing to stay aware of your emotions, both positive and negative?

DAY FOUR: In what ways have you most significantly changed spiritually? How has your relationship with God deepened? How has drawing closer to Him made a difference in the other three areas of your life?

DAY FIVE: In what ways have you most significantly changed physically? Have you met or exceeded your weight/measurement goals? How has your health improved?

DAY SIX: Was there one person in your First Place for Health group who was particularly encouraging to you? How did their kindness make a difference in your First Place for Health journey?

DAY SEVEN: Summarize the previous six questions into a one-page testimony, or "faith story," to share at your group's victory celebration.

"Now may our Lord Jesus Christ Himself and God our Father, who loved us and by His grace gave us eternal comfort and a wonderful hope, comfort you and strengthen you in every good thing you do and say." (2 Thessalonians 2:16-17)

LEADER DISCUSSION GUIDE

For in-depth information, guidance and helpful tips about leading a successful First Place for Health group, spend time studying the *My Place for Leadership* book. In it, you will find valuable answers to most of your questions, as well as personal insights from many First Place for Health group leaders.

For the group meetings in this session, be sure to read and consider each week's discussion topics several days before the meeting—some questions and activities require supplies and/or planning to complete. Also, if you are leading a large group, plan to break into smaller groups for discussion and then come together as a large group to share your answers and responses. Make sure to appoint a capable leader for each small group so that discussions stay focused and on track (and be sure each group records their answers!).

—— WEEK ONE: GRACE TO SAY YES

1. Do you see yourself as an athlete? Have you ever competed in a race or other athletic activity? How has our study this week influenced your perspective?
2. On Day 1 you were asked to write down your "Why"—as in "Why did you sign up for this study? Why are you running this race? What is your motivation?" Share that with our group.
3. You were also asked what makes you anxious, worried, or afraid. Be brave and share these answers, too, so that we can support and encourage you.
4. What encouragement did you find in the verses we read this week? Did you have a favorite? Is there one that stood out to you?
5. On Day 2 we talked about the race of faith being so much bigger than our battle to lose weight (see Romans 8:29-30). Why is this important to remember? Where does our health and wellness journey fit into all of this? What connections did you make?
6. In Ephesians 3:14-20 (see Day 3) we learned that we have the power to be all that God created us to be and do all that He created us to do. Where does this power come from? How do we access it or experience it? How do we know it's powerful enough?
7. Share one specific goal you set on Day 4 and the step that you will take to reach it over the next eight weeks.
8. What are some of the practical steps you've been taking so that you are prepared and equipped to "run to win" this race? (See Day 5.)

9. On Day 6 you designed a race bib and wrote out your race strategy. Share one or both with the group.
10. What glimpses of grace did God give you this week?

—— WEEK TWO: GRACE TO SAY NO

1. On Day 1, what image comes to mind when you think about how you're running your race this week? Why do you think it's important to distinguish between a symptom of sin (like overeating) and the root cause of it? What encouragement did you find in the Scriptures you read?
2. What are some of the lesser things, the "permissible but not beneficial" things you identified on Day 2—and how have they been hindering you? How can you say "no" to or "throw off" those things?
3. Why do you think doubt and double-mindedness are so crippling (Day 3)? What role can accountability play here? What else can you do to strengthen your confidence and resolve—particularly in regard to your health and wellness?
4. What kind of impact does negativity (grumbling and complaining) have on our physical, mental, emotional, and spiritual well-being (Day 4)? How does it hinder us in our race?
5. What five things did you find in Colossians 3:16-17 that can turn around our attitudes?
6. Share some of your responses to the "have to/get to" exercise.
7. On Day 5, we looked at the impact of unhealthy or destructive desires. What kinds of desires relate to our health and wellness journey?
8. Where or how have you experienced the promise of Philippians 2:13 (God's power at work) in your life in the past? Where do you need it now?
9. If you're willing to share, what words or phrases in the Liturgy jumped out at you? Why? Take a few moments to pray this prayer out loud together as a group. Allow for a brief period of silence and contemplation.
10. What glimpses of grace did God give you this week?

—— WEEK THREE: GRACE TO HOLD ON

1. Have you ever thought of Jesus as your Coach or Personal Trainer? What difference does it make that He was (and is) fully God and fully man? How has He been coaching you this week?
2. What did you learn (remember) about who Jesus is and what He has done on Day 1? How is He truly our "all-purpose answer"? How have you experienced His help as you run your race?
3. How do the verses we read on Day 2 help us better understand our memory verse? What are we looking to Jesus for—and why? And why is it so important?

4. What did you think of Jane Rubietta's description of the love with which Jesus looks at us (Day 2)? Is that hard for you to believe? Why or why not?

5. Which of the promises on Day 3 was most meaningful to you this week?

6. What are the differences among physical, emotional, and spiritual hunger (Day 3)? How does Jesus meet each of these needs? Have you experienced Him as "more satisfying than the most delicious feast"? In what way?

7. Which of the "hold on" verses on Day 4 spoke to you—and why?

8. There's so much powerful imagery in the verses we read at the end of Day 5. We can picture ourselves and our loved ones as Jesus's little lambs, being held in His arms, held "close to His heart," or held in His hands. Which of these images resonated most with you? Did you write a prayer or draw a hand—and if you, did, how did it help you?

9. What practical steps did you take to help you keep your eyes on Jesus (Day 6)?

10. What glimpses of grace did God give you this week?

—— WEEK FOUR: GRACE TO LET GO

1. In the introduction to this week, we talked about five mindsets that can trip us up. Which one(s) resonated with you? Are there others that you thought of?

2. On Day 1, we talked about God as our Way Maker. How have you experienced this? What "impossible" things has He done for you in the past or is He doing now?

3. What's the difference between our common understanding of "perfection" and the biblical use of that word (Day 2)? Practically speaking, how can we resist unhealthy perfectionism and focus on progress, growth, and maturity instead?

4. Can you think of some examples of all-or-nothing thinking that sabotage you (Day 2)? What can you replace them with? What can you say to yourself instead?

5. What did we learn on Day 3 about God's heart toward us? (See Isaiah 40:11, Matthew 11:28-30, and Colossians 3:12-13.)

6. Is it hard for you to be kind to yourself? Why is it necessary? What can you do to practice kindness to yourself and other runners in this race?

7. How can comparison and competition become unhealthy? How can it be a distraction? What's a better way to run this race? (See Day 4.)

8. On Day 5 we talked about "growing slow." How do you respond to that idea? What have you learned about God's timing? What do you think it means to wait "hopefully and expectantly"?

9. Re-read the balloon story on Day 6. On a piece of paper, draw the shape of a balloon or several balloons. Inside, write down whatever (or whoever) you need to give to Jesus today. Take a few moments right now to release them in prayer.

10. What glimpses of grace did God give you this week?

—— WEEK FIVE: GRACE TO LEARN AND GROW

1. Do you have a favorite movie with the kind of montage we talked about in the Introduction to this week? How about a favorite workout song or playlist? What motivates, inspires, and energizes you?

2. What have you learned from your victories (Day 1)? What are your top tips or go-to strategies?

3. What have you learned from your defeats (Day 2)? How have they been helpful to you? (Note that the questions on Day 1 and Day 2 could also function as a midway goal check: consider what's going well and not going well in each area, and make adjustments.)

4. Who is on your support team? Whom are you supporting (Day 3)? What role does your First Place for Health group play? What have you learned from your participation with this group?

5. On Day 4 we talked about learning from our weaknesses. Is it hard for you to acknowledge and accept your weaknesses? Why or why not?

6. Which of the verses on Day 4 was most meaningful to you?

7. How have you learned to lean on God's strength (Day 5)? What does that mean, practically speaking? What does it look like for you?

8. Have you ever battled "Esau Syndrome" (Day 5)? What has helped you?

9. On Day 6 we talked about rest and Sabbath-keeping as a necessary part of our training. Why do you think it's so important? Is resting hard or easy for you? Why? What refreshes and recharges you?

10. What glimpses of grace did God give you this week?

—— WEEK SIX: GRACE TO BELIEVE

1. How are discipline and correction part of our training program for greater health and wellness and for our race of faith? Why is it not punishment? What's the difference?

2. When we talk about God's discipline or correction, why do we need to start by reflecting on His character? What did you learn about that this week? Share your affirmation or prayer from Day 1. What is your testimony?

3. What was your favorite Scripture from Day 2? How or why did this specific verse speak to you?

4. On Day 2 we talked about resisting discipline vs. responding to discipline. How would you describe the difference? Ideally, how should we respond to discipline or correction? Why?

5. How can we come to see pain or adversity as a gift (Day 3)? Read 2 Corinthians 4:17. How can you relate this to your health and wellness journey? How would you put it in your own words?

6. Read aloud the FCA Creed quoted on Day 4. How might this kind of approach

or perspective be game-changing—particularly when it comes to our health and wellness?

7. What is God calling you to sacrifice or surrender and what does that look like?

8. Conversations about discipline and correction and sacrifice can be heavy. What hope or encouragement did you find in this week's study? Did anything from Day 5 resonate with you?

9. Read Psalm 103:7-14 from Day 2 and Micah 7:18-20. Share some of the things you wrote on Day 6 that have been swept into the sea—and celebrate that!

10. What glimpses of grace did God give you this week?

—— WEEK SEVEN: GRACE TO RECEIVE

1. This week we're talking about temptation. How have you approached your battles with temptation in the past? How (where) have you been successful or unsuccessful?

2. How might seeing temptation as an opportunity be a game-changer? What is it an opportunity for? (There's more than one answer!)

3. What worldly sources of temptation did you identify on Day 1? What does Jesus promise in John 16:33? How might you apply this to your health and wellness journey?

4. On Day 2 we talked about being our own worst enemy. How have you experienced that? Re-read the quote from Philip Graham Ryken. How does it help to be aware of when we are most vulnerable to temptation? How can we let our battles drive us to prayer and not to despair?

5. On Day 3 we talked about our enemy, the devil. Why do you think he has made our health and wellness such a battleground? Why does he come after us physically, mentally, emotionally, and spiritually? How are these temptations related to one another?

6. How do we pray "Thy will, not my will" when it comes to our health and wellness (Day 4)? How can we resist temptation, as Jesus did? What can we learn from Him?

7. Share your own prayer from Day 4.

8. What wisdom or insight did you gain from the brainstorming exercise on Day 5? What plan did you come up with? Have you had a chance to put it into practice? What happened?

9. What saying did you choose for your sign on Day 6? Why? What does it mean to you? Whom did you choose to share it with?

10. What glimpses of grace did God give you this week?

—— WEEK EIGHT: GRACE TO GO THE DISTANCE

1. .How are you feeling as you run your race today? Where are you physically, mentally, emotionally, spiritually? (Pick one to share.)

2. What tempts you to "grow weary" — to want to give up and give in? What are some of the obstacles you're facing right now?

3. On Day 2, we talked about encouraging others as a way to combat our own discouragement. Have you tried that? What did you do? How did it work?

4. Carol Kent talked about God being our "only true Rock." (Day 3). Read Psalm 18:2, Psalm 31:2-4, and Psalm 62:5-8. How do these verses speak to you?

5. What are some of the obstacles you have already overcome? (Day 4) How did you do it? How did God bring you through it?

6. Read Paul's race strategies in Philippians 4:6-9. Which of these have you put into practice? How have they worked for you?

7. Why do you think Philippians 4:8 is such an important strategy? Can you relate this to your health and wellness journey?

8. We looked at three "calls to persevere" on Day 5. Which one resonates most with you — and why?

9. Take turns reading aloud Paul's Pep Talk from Day 6. What struck you most? Anything you would add?

10. What glimpses of grace did God give you this week?

—— WEEK NINE: TIME TO CELEBRATE

Most of your meeting this week will be a victory celebration. (See "Planning a Victory Celebration" in My Place for Leadership.) Be sure to take some time at the beginning of the meeting to talk about how much it has meant to you to lead the study, how much you appreciate each person's presence and participation, how much God loves each person in the group, and how faithful He is to give us grace for the race.

For the rest of the study time, invite each member to tell his or her Grace for the Race story. Ask them where they have seen—or been most aware of—God's grace this session.

In a very real sense, your race isn't over yet—not until you run into the arms of Jesus! So be sure to talk about your group's future plans, and make each person feel welcome to continue on with you.

End your celebration by reading aloud this Scripture-based benediction: "May the grace of our Lord Jesus—His favor, His blessing, His presence—go with you and remain with you, now and always!"

FIRST PLACE FOR HEALTH
JUMP START MENUS

All recipe and menu nutritional information was determined using the Master-Cook software, a program that accesses a database containing more than 6,000 food items prepared using the United States Department of Agriculture (USDA) publications and information from food manufacturers.

As with any nutritional program, MasterCook calculates the nutritional values of the recipes based on ingredients. Nutrition may vary due to how the food is prepared, where the food comes from, soil content, season, ripeness, processing and method of preparation. You are expected to add snacks and sides as needed to meet your nutritional needs. For these reasons, please use the recipes and menu plans as approximate guides. As always, consult your physician and/or a registered dietitian before starting a weight-loss program.

Apple and Sweet Potato Mini Muffins

Nonstick cooking spray
10 slices Canadian bacon
2 cups chopped apples
½ cup chopped onion
1 medium sweet potato, peeled and cut into ¼-inch pieces
½ teaspoon dried thyme, crushed
¼ teaspoon black pepper
6 eggs, lightly beaten
¾ cup fat-free milk
¾ cup shredded reduced-fat cheddar cheese

Preheat oven to 350o. Coat twelve muffin cups with cooking spray. Cut four of the bacon slices into three pieces; chop remaining bacon. In a skillet cook large bacon pieces over medium until crisp. Drain bacon on paper towels; discard drippings. Add chopped bacon, apples, and onion to skillet. Cook over medium heat for 5 minutes, stirring occasionally. Add sweet potato; cook 10 minutes or until potato is tender, stirring frequently. Stir in thyme and pepper. Divide potato mixture among prepared muffin cups. In a medium bowl combine egg and milk; pour over potato mixture (cups will be full). Top with cheese. Bake 25 minutes or until puffed and a knife comes out clean. Cool in cups 5 minutes. Remove from cups. Top with large bacon pieces. Serve warm. Serves 6

Nutritional Information: 198 Calories, 6g Fat, 22g Carbohydrates, 15g Protein, 3g Fiber, 16mg Cholesterol, 387mg Sodium

Cucumber-Chicken Wrap

1 ounce cream cheese, at room temperature
¼ medium avocado, mashed
1 teaspoon lemon juice
⅛ teaspoon salt
⅛ teaspoon ground pepper
2 tablespoons chopped fresh dill
1 (8 inch) whole-wheat tortilla
¼ cup shredded cooked chicken
2 tablespoons shredded carrot
6 thin slices cucumber
½ cup mixed salad greens

Stir cream cheese, avocado, lemon juice, salt and pepper together in a small bowl. Add dill and stir until well blended. Spread the mixture evenly on tortilla. Top with chicken, carrot, cucumber and greens, then roll up like a burrito. Serves 1

Nutritional Information: 353 Calories, 19g Fat, 28g Carbohydrates, 18g Protein, 6g Fiber, 18g Protein, 58mg Cholesterol, 590mg Sodium

Stuffed Pepper Casserole

2 tablespoons extra-virgin olive oil

1 pound 90%-lean ground beef

1 large red onion, thinly sliced

3 medium red and yellow bell peppers, thinly sliced

6 cloves garlic, chopped

2 teaspoons paprika

2 teaspoons dried oregano

1 teaspoon salt

¾ teaspoon ground pepper

2 tablespoons tomato paste

1 (14.5 ounce) can no-salt-added fire-roasted diced tomatoes, drained

1 (8.8-ounce) package cooked brown rice

½ cup unsalted beef broth

1 cup shredded low-moisture part-skim mozzarella cheese

Preheat oven to 400°F. Heat oil in a large nonstick skillet over medium heat. Add beef; cook, stirring often and breaking up beef, until cooked through and no longer pink, about 5 minutes. Add onion, bell peppers, garlic, paprika, oregano, salt and pepper; cook, stirring often, until the vegetables are tender, about 8 minutes. Increase heat to medium-high and stir in tomato paste; cook, stirring constantly, until the paste darkens, about 1 minute. Remove from heat. Stir in drained tomatoes, rice and broth.

Transfer the mixture to a 9-by-13-inch baking dish; cover with foil. Bake until the rice is tender, about 20 minutes. Uncover and sprinkle evenly with cheese. Bake, uncovered, until the cheese is melted and beginning to bubble, about 10 minutes. Serves 6

Nutritional Information: 344 Calories, 17g Fat, 24g Carbohydrates, 23g Protein, 4g Fiber, 61mg Cholesterol, Sodium 610mg

Southwestern-style Waffle

1 frozen whole-grain waffle, such as Van's 8 Whole Grains Multigrain
1 egg, cooked sunny-side up
¼ medium avocado, halved, seeded, peeled and chopped
1 tablespoon refrigerated fresh salsa

Toast waffle according to package directions. Top with egg, avocado, and salsa.
Serves 1

Nutritional Information: 207 Calories, 12g Fat, 17g Carbohydrate, 9g Protein,
6g Fiber, 185mg Cholesterol, 279mg Sodium

Chopped Salad with Peanut Dressing

1 10-ounce package kale, Brussels sprout, broccoli and cabbage salad mix
1 12-ounce package frozen shelled edamame, thawed
2 7-ounce packages Sriracha-flavored baked tofu, cubed
1/2 cup spicy peanut vinaigrette from your favorite store

Divide salad mix among four bowls. Top each with 1/2 cup edamame and one-fourth of the tofu. Dress with vinaigrette up to 1 day before serving. Serves 4

Nutritional Information: 332 Calories, 15g Fat, 26g Carbohydrates, 27g Protein, 8g Fiber, 27g Protein, Sodium 236mg

Skillet Ravioli Lasagna

1 24-ounce package frozen or refrigerated cheese ravioli
1 pound lean ground beef
1 ½ teaspoons dried oregano
½ teaspoon garlic powder
½ teaspoon salt
¼ teaspoon ground pepper
1 28-ounce can no-salt-added crushed tomatoes
¼ cup chopped fresh basil
8 ounces small fresh mozzarella balls, divided

Preheat broiler. Cook ravioli according to package directions; drain and set aside. Meanwhile, cook ground beef in a large broiler-safe skillet over medium-high heat until cooked through, 4 to 5 minutes. Season with oregano, garlic powder, salt and pepper. Add tomatoes and basil; bring to a simmer. Fold in the cooked ravioli and half of the mozzarella balls.

Scatter the remaining mozzarella balls over the top of the pasta. Carefully transfer the pan to the oven. Broil until the cheese is melted, 2 to 3 minutes. Serves 6

Nutritional Information: 483 Calories, 20g Fat, 34g Carbohydrates, 38g Protein, 3g Fiber, 127mg Cholesterol, Sodium 630mg

Banana-Blueberry Muffins

¾ cup whole-wheat flour
¾ cup all-purpose flour
1 teaspoon baking soda
1 teaspoon baking powder
¾ teaspoon ground cinnamon
½ teaspoon salt
¼ teaspoon ground ginger
2 medium bananas, mashed (about 1 cup)
⅓ cup honey
⅓ cup cottage cheese
¼ cup smooth natural peanut butter
¼ cup reduced-fat milk
1 large egg
1 ½ teaspoons vanilla extract
2 cups fresh or frozen blueberries

Preheat oven to 350°F. Coat a 12-cup muffin tin with cooking spray. Whisk whole-wheat flour, all-purpose flour, baking soda, baking powder, cinnamon, salt and ginger together in a medium bowl until combined. Place mashed bananas, honey, cottage cheese, peanut butter, milk, egg and vanilla in a large bowl; beat with an electric mixer on medium speed until well combined, about 1 minute. Add the flour mixture; beat on low speed until just combined and a thick batter forms, about 45 seconds. Using a rubber spatula, gently fold in blueberries until evenly distributed. Spoon the batter into the prepared muffin cups, about 1/3 cup each. Bake until golden and a wooden pick inserted in the centers comes out clean, 18 to 22 minutes. Let cool in the pan for 5 minutes before transferring to a wire rack. Serve warm or at room temperature. Serves 12

To Store: Store in an airtight container at room temperature for up to 1 week or wrap and freeze for up to 3 months.

Nutritional Information: 166 Calories, 4g Fat, 29g Carbohydrate, 5g Protein, 17mg Cholesterol, 292mg Sodium

Quick Tuna Melt

1 5-ounce can no-salt-added water-packed tuna, drained
1 small celery stalk, chopped
2 tablespoons chopped jarred roasted red pepper
1 scallion, minced
3 tablespoons low-fat plain Greek yogurt
1 teaspoon Dijon mustard
¼ teaspoon ground pepper
4 teaspoons mayonnaise
4 slices whole-grain bread
2 slices sharp Cheddar cheese

Stir tuna, celery, roasted red pepper, scallion, yogurt, mustard and pepper together in a medium bowl until well blended. Spread 1 teaspoon mayonnaise on
one side of each slice of bread. Flip 2 of the slices and top each with half of the
tuna mixture, 1 slice cheese and another slice of bread, mayonnaise-side up.
Heat a large skillet over medium heat. Place the sandwiches in the pan and cook,
turning once, until the cheese is melted and the bread is golden, 3 to 5 minutes
per side. Serve immediately. Serves 1

Nutritional Information: 382 Calories, 13g Fat, 29g Carbohydrates, 34g Protein, 50mg Cholesterol, 675mg Sodium

Chicken Cutlets with Sun-Dried Tomato Cream Sauce

1 pound chicken cutlets
¼ teaspoon salt, divided
¼ teaspoon ground pepper, divided
½ cup oil-packed sun-dried tomatoes, plus 1 tablespoon oil from the jar
½ cup finely chopped shallots
½ cup chicken broth
½ cup heavy cream
2 tablespoons chopped fresh parsley

Sprinkle chicken with 1/8 teaspoon each salt and pepper. Heat sun-dried tomato oil in a large skillet over medium heat. Add the chicken and cook, turning once, until browned and an instant-read thermometer inserted into the thickest part registers 165°F, about 6 minutes total. Transfer to a plate. Add sun-dried tomatoes and shallots to the pan. Cook, stirring, for 1 minute. Increase heat to high and add wine. Cook, scraping up any browned bits, until the liquid has mostly evaporated, about 2 minutes. Reduce heat to medium and stir in cream, any accumulated juices from the chicken and the remaining 1/8 teaspoon each salt and pepper; simmer for 2 minutes. Return the chicken to the pan and turn to coat with the sauce. Serve the chicken topped with the sauce and parsley. Serves 4

Nutritional Information: 324 Calories, 19g Fat, 8g Carbohydrates, 25gProtein, 97mg Cholesterol, 1g Fiber, Sodium 250mg

Parmesan Eggs

4 large eggs, yolks and whites separated
Pinch of salt
¼ cup finely grated Parmesan cheese
1 scallion, finely chopped
Ground pepper to taste

Preheat oven to 450 degrees F. Line a large baking sheet with parchment paper. Lightly coat with cooking spray. Separate egg whites from the yolks, placing each yolk in an individual small bowl. Beat all of the egg whites and salt in a mixing bowl with an electric mixer on high speed until stiff. Gently fold Parmesan and scallions into the beaten whites with a rubber spatula. Make 4 mounds (about 3/4 cup each) of egg-cheese mixture on the prepared baking sheet. Make a well in the middle of each mound with the back of a spoon.

Bake the egg whites until starting to lightly brown, about 3 minutes. Remove from oven. If the well has filled in during baking, use the spoon to recreate it. Gently slip a yolk into each well. Bake until the yolks are cooked but still runny, 3 to 5 minutes more. Sprinkle with pepper. Serve immediately. Serves 4

Nutritional Information: 94 Calories, 6g Fat, 1g Carbohydrates, 8g Protein, 0g Fiber, 190mg Cholesterol, 198mg Sodium

Roasted Veggie & Quinoa Salad

2 cups mixed salad greens
1 cup roasted vegetables
½ cup cooked quinoa
1-2 tablespoons vinaigrette (see recipe)
1 tablespoon crumbled feta cheese
1 tablespoon sunflower seeds

Combine greens, roasted vegetables and quinoa; drizzle with vinaigrette. Top the salad with feta and sunflower seeds. Serves 1

Nutritional Information: 351 Calories, 18g Fat, 39g Carbohydrates, 10g Protein, 8mg Cholesterol, 381mg Sodium

Herb Vinaigrette

⅓ cup extra-virgin olive oil
⅓ cup rice vinegar
1 tablespoon dried oregano
2 tablespoons finely chopped shallots
2 tablespoons lemon juice
¼ teaspoon salt
¼ teaspoon ground pepper

Combine oil, vinegar, herbs, shallot, lime (or lemon) juice, salt and pepper in a jar with a tight-fitting lid. Cover and shake until well combined. Refrigerate for up to 5 days. Shake well before serving.

Nutritional Information: (2 tablespoons): 78 Calories, 8g Fat, 1g Carbohydrates, 66mg Sodium

Creamy Chicken Noodle Soup with Rotisserie Chicken

2 tablespoons unsalted butter
1 tablespoon olive oil
2 cups chopped yellow onion
1 cup chopped carrots
1 cup chopped celery
1 ¾ teaspoons kosher salt
3 tablespoons all-purpose flour
4 cups unsalted chicken stock
2 cups whole milk
4 ounces uncooked whole-wheat egg noodles
3 cups coarsely chopped rotisserie chicken breast
1 cup frozen green peas

Melt butter with olive oil in a large Dutch oven over medium-high heat. Add onion, carrots, celery and salt and cook, stirring often, until vegetables are slightly softened, 6 to 8 minutes. Add flour and stir to coat. Stir in stock and milk and let the mixture come to a boil. Add uncooked noodles to the boiling mixture. Cover and cook until noodles are al dente, about 8 minutes. Stir in chicken and peas and cook until pasta reaches desired doneness and chicken and peas are warmed through, about 1 to 2 more minutes. Serve immediately. Serves 8

Nutritional Information: 258 Calories, 9g Fat, 24g Carbohydrates, 23g Protein, 4g Fiber, Sodium 730mg

Sweet Potato Toast with Spinach & Egges

1 large slice sweet potato (1/4 inch thick)
⅓ cup cooked spinach
1 large egg, fried or poached
½ teaspoon sliced fresh chives
½ teaspoon hot sauce

Toast sweet potato in a toaster or toaster oven until just cooked through and starting to brown, 12 to 15 minutes. Top with spinach, egg, chives and hot sauce. Serves 1

Nutritional Information: 124 Calories, 5g Fat, 12g Carbohydrate, 9g Protein, 186mg Cholesterol, 190mg Sodium

3-Ingredient Chicken Salad Tostadas

1 10-ounce Southwest-style salad kit
6 ounces rotisserie chicken breast, shredded
6 tostada shells

Prepare salad kit according to package directions, reserving tortilla strips and shredded cheese; fold in chicken. Divide the chicken salad mixture among tostada shells. Top with the reserved tortilla strips and cheese. Serves 2

Nutritional Information: 437 Calories, 21g Fat, 33g Carbohydrates, 30g Protein, 5g Fiber, 855mg Sodium

Lemon Chicken Skillet

12 ounces small red potatoes, halved
1 tablespoon olive oil, divided
4 6-ounce skinless, boneless chicken breast halves, pounded to 3/4-inch thickness
¾ teaspoon kosher salt, divided
½ teaspoon freshly ground black pepper, divided
4 ounces mushrooms, quartered
1 tablespoon chopped fresh thyme or 1 tsp dried
¼ cup whole milk
5 teaspoons all-purpose flour
1 ¾ cups unsalted chicken stock
8 very thin lemon slices
1 8-ounce package trimmed green beans
2 tablespoons chopped fresh flat-leaf parsley

Preheat oven to 450°F. Place potatoes in a medium saucepan; cover with water. Bring to a boil, and simmer 12 minutes or until tender. Drain. Heat a large ovenproof skillet over medium-high heat. Add 1 teaspoon oil to pan. Sprinkle chicken with 1/4 teaspoon salt and 1/4 teaspoon pepper. Add chicken to pan; cook 5 minutes or until chicken is browned. Turn chicken over. Place pan in oven; bake at 450°F for 10 minutes or until chicken is done. Remove chicken from pan.
Return pan to medium-high heat. Add remaining 2 teaspoons oil. Add potatoes, cut sides down; mushrooms; and thyme; cook 3 minutes or until browned, stirring once. Combine milk and flour in a small bowl, stirring with a whisk. Add remaining salt, remaining pepper, flour mixture, stock, lemon, and beans to pan; simmer 1 minute or until slightly thickened. Add chicken; cover, reduce heat, and simmer 3 minutes or until beans are crisp-tender. Sprinkle with parsley. Serves 4

Nutritional Information: 342 Calories, 9g Fat, 23g Carbohydrates, 43g Protein, 4g Fiber, 110mg Cholesterol, Sodium 642mg

Peanut Butter-Chocolate Chip Oatmeal Muffins

3 cups old-fashioned rolled oats
1 ½ cups low-fat milk
½ cup creamy natural peanut butter, divided
¼ cup unsweetened applesauce
2 large eggs, lightly beaten
3 tablespoons packed light brown sugar
1 teaspoon baking powder
1 teaspoon vanilla extract
½ teaspoon salt
¼ cup mini semisweet chocolate chips

Preheat oven to 375°F. Coat a 12-cup muffin tin with cooking spray. Combine oats, milk, 1/4 cup peanut butter, applesauce, eggs, brown sugar, baking powder, vanilla and salt in a large bowl. Fill each muffin cup with a heaping 2 tablespoons of batter, then divide the remaining 1/4 cup peanut butter and chocolate chips among the muffin cups, about 1 teaspoon each. Cover with the remaining batter, about 2 tablespoons each. Bake until a toothpick inserted in the center comes out clean, about 25 minutes. Cool in the pan for 10 minutes, then turn out onto a wire rack. Serve warm or at room temperature. Serves 12

Nutritional Information: 204 Calories, 9g Fat, 24g Carbohydrates, 7g Protein, 33mg Cholesterol, 199mg Sodium

Fruit & Cheese Bento Box

2 or 3 whole-grain crispbreads or 6 whole-grain crackers
1 ounce Cheddar cheese, cubed or sliced
1 ounce goat cheese
¼ cup smoked almonds
½ apple, sliced
1 tablespoon fig jam
½ large carrot, peeled and cut into 4-inch sticks

Arrange crispbreads (or crackers), Cheddar, goat cheese, almonds, apple, jam and carrot sticks in a 4-cup divided sealable container (Can be separated with cupcake liners, if needed) Keep refrigerated until ready to eat. Serves 1

Nutritional Information: 557 Calories, 35g Fat, 45g Carbohydrates, 21g Protein, 41mg Cholesterol, 528mg Sodium

Chicken Parmesan Casserole

    8 ounces whole-wheat rotini
    4 tablespoons extra-virgin olive oil, divided
    1 cup chopped onion
    1 28-ounce can no-salt-added crushed tomatoes
    1 teaspoon garlic powder
    ½ teaspoon dried basil
    ½ teaspoon dried oregano
    ½ teaspoon salt
    ¼ teaspoon crushed red pepper
    2 cups shredded cooked chicken
    1 cup shredded mozzarella cheese
    ½ cup panko breadcrumbs
    ¼ cup grated Parmesan cheese
    2 tablespoons chopped parsley

Preheat oven to 400 degrees F. Lightly coat an 8-inch-square baking dish with cooking spray. Bring a large saucepan of water to a boil. Add rotini and cook according to package directions. Drain. Meanwhile, heat 2 tablespoons oil in a large skillet over medium heat. Add onion and cook, stirring, until starting to soften, about 3 minutes. Add tomatoes, garlic powder, basil, oregano, salt and crushed red pepper; bring to a simmer. Cook, stirring, until thickened, about 5 minutes. Stir in chicken and the cooked rotini. Transfer to the prepared baking dish and top with mozzarella. Stir panko, Parmesan, parsley and the remaining 2 tablespoons oil together in a small bowl. Sprinkle over the casserole. Bake until hot and the topping is golden, 25 to 30 minutes. Serves 6

Nutritional Information: 442 Calories, 17g Fat, 50g Carbohydrates, 26g Protein, 9g Fiber, 43mg Cholesterol, Sodium 462mg

Cinnamon Pear Muffinsg

Nonstick cooking spray
1 cup all-purpose flour
½ cup whole wheat flour
1 ½ teaspoons baking powder
1 teaspoon ground cinnamon
½ teaspoon baking soda
½ teaspoon ground ginger
¼ teaspoon salt
¼ teaspoon ground nutmeg
1 egg, lightly beaten
1 cup buttermilk
⅔ cup packed brown sugar (see Tips)
⅓ cup canola oil
2 teaspoons vanilla
2 medium pears
2 teaspoons lemon juice
1 teaspoon powdered sugar

Preheat oven to 400 degrees F. Coat eighteen 2 1/2-inch muffin cups with cooking spray. In a medium bowl combine the next eight ingredients (through nutmeg). Make a well in center of mixture. In a small bowl combine the next five ingredients (through vanilla). Add to flour mixture; stir just until moistened.

Peel pears. Cut 18 thin pear slices and brush with lemon juice. Chop all of the remaining pear and fold into batter. Spoon batter into prepared muffin cups. Top with pear slices. Bake on separate oven racks 18 to 20 minutes or until a toothpick comes out clean, switching positions of pans halfway through baking. Immediately remove from cups; cool on wire racks. Dust with powdered sugar. Serves 18

Nutritional Information: 127 Calories, 5g Fat, 20g Carbohydrates, 2g Protein, 11g Cholesterol, 129mg Sodium

Crispy Chickpea Bowl with Lemon Vinaigrette

⅔ cup quinoa

1 ⅓ cups water plus 1 tablespoon, divided

⅛ teaspoon salt plus 1/4 teaspoon, divided

1 15-ounce can no-salt-added chickpeas, rinsed

1 small red onion, thinly sliced

4 teaspoons extra-virgin olive oil plus 2 tablespoons, divided

¼ teaspoon ground pepper, divided

1 bunch kale, stems removed, thinly sliced (about 5 cups)

1 teaspoon Dijon mustard

1 clove garlic, minced

2 teaspoons lemon zest

2 tablespoons lemon juice

1 red bell pepper, thinly sliced

¼ cup crumbled feta cheese

2 tablespoons toasted pumpkin seeds

Preheat oven to 400 degrees F. Coat a large rimmed baking sheet liberally with cooking spray. Combine quinoa, 1 1/3 cups water, and 1/8 teaspoon salt in a medium saucepan. Bring to a boil over medium-high heat. Reduce heat to medium-low, partially cover, and simmer until the quinoa is tender, about 15 minutes. Drain any excess water. Meanwhile, pat chickpeas dry with a paper towel. Toss with onion, 2 teaspoons oil, and 1/8 teaspoon each salt and pepper in a large bowl. Spread out on the prepared baking sheet. Roast for 15 minutes. Toss kale with 2 teaspoons oil and the remaining 1/8 teaspoon salt in the large bowl. Stir the kale into the chickpeas and roast for 15 minutes more. Whisk mustard, garlic, lemon zest, lemon juice, the remaining 1 tablespoon water and the remaining 1/8 teaspoon pepper in a small bowl. Whisk in the remaining 2 tablespoons oil. Divide the quinoa among 4 serving bowls. Top with the kale mixture, bell pepper slices, feta, and pumpkin seeds. Drizzle with the vinaigrette. Serves 4

Nutritional Information: 370 Calories, 18g Fat, 41g Carbohydrates, 12g Protein, 9g Fiber, 8mg Cholesterol, Sodium 486mg

Easy Chicken Enchilada Casserole

2 tablespoons extra-virgin olive oil

4 bell peppers, sliced

3 cups sliced sweet onions

1 teaspoon salt

1 28-ounce can crushed tomatoes

2 tablespoons ground cumin

1/2-1 teaspoon ground chipotle Chile powder

¼ teaspoon salt

8 corn tortillas, cut into wedges

1 15-ounce can black beans, rinsed and drained

1 cup chopped roasted Chicken Thighs (see recipe)

1 ½ cups shredded Mexican cheese blend (6 ounces), divided

Heat oil in a large skillet or Dutch oven over medium heat. Add peppers, onions and salt; cook, stirring occasionally, until the vegetables are tender and starting to brown, 18 to 21 minutes. Stir tomatoes, cumin, chili powder and salt together in a medium bowl. Coat an 8-by-11" casserole dish with cooking spray. Spoon 1/2 cup of the tomato sauce into the bottom of the prepared dish. Arrange 1/3 of the tortilla wedges over the tomato sauce. Top with half of the beans, half of the chicken and half of the pepper mixture. Top with 1 cup sauce and 1/2 cup cheese. Layer on half the remaining tortillas. Top with the remaining beans, chicken and pepper mixture. Top with 1 cup of the sauce and 1/2 cup cheese. Layer on the remaining tortillas, followed by the remaining sauce (about 1/3 cup). Sprinkle with the remaining 1/2 cup cheese. Preheat oven to 375°. Bake the casserole, uncovered, until hot and bubbling, 35 to 40 minutes. Serves 6

Nutritional Information: 365 Calories, 15g Fat, 39g Carbohydrates, 21g Protein, 9g Fiber, 49mg Cholesterol, Sodium 770mg

Roasted Chicken Thighs

1 ¾ pounds boneless, skinless chicken thighs, trimmed

2 teaspoons extra-virgin olive oil

1 large clove garlic, minced

1 teaspoon kosher salt & 1 teaspoon dried oregano

Preheat oven to 425o. Line a baking sheet with parchment paper. Place chicken in a large bowl. Add oil, garlic, salt and oregano; toss until well coated. Arrange the chicken on the prepared pan. Roast until cooked through, 18 to 22 minutes. Serves 6

STEPS FOR SPIRITUAL GROWTH

—— GOD'S WORD FOR YOUR LIFE

I have hidden your word in my heart that I might not sin against you. Psalm 119:11

As you begin to make decisions based on what God's Word teaches you, you will want to memorize what He has promised to those who trust and follow Him. Second Peter 1:3 tells us that God "has given us everything we need for life and godliness through our knowledge of him" (emphasis added). The Bible provides instruction and encouragement for any area of life in which you may be struggling. If you are dealing with a particular emotion or traumatic life event—fear, discouragement, stress, financial upset, the death of a loved one, a relationship difficulty—you can search through a Bible concordance for Scripture passages that deal with that particular situation. Scripture provides great comfort to those who memorize it.

One of the promises of knowing and obeying God's Word is that it gives you wisdom, insight, and understanding above all worldly knowledge (see Psalm 119:97–104). Psalm 119:129–130 says, "Your statutes are wonderful; therefore I obey them. The unfolding of your words gives light; it gives understanding to the simple." Now that's a precious promise about guidance for life!

The Value of Scripture Memory

Scripture memory is an important part of the Christian life. There are four key reasons to memorize Scripture:

TO HANDLE DIFFICULT SITUATIONS. A heartfelt knowledge of God's Word will equip you to handle any situation that you might face. Declaring such truth as, "I can do everything through Christ" (see Philippians 4:13) and "he will never leave me or forsake me" (see Hebrews 13:5) will enable you to walk through situations with peace and courage.

TO OVERCOME TEMPTATION. Luke 4:1–13 describes how Jesus used Scripture to overcome His temptations in the desert (see also Matthew 4:1-11). Knowledge of Scripture and the strength that comes with the ability to use it are important parts of putting on the full armor of God in preparation for spiritual warfare (see Ephesians 6:10–18).

TO GET GUIDANCE. Psalm 119:105 states the Word of God "is a lamp to my feet and a light for my path." You learn to hide God's Word in your heart so His light will direct your decisions and actions throughout your day.

TO TRANSFORM YOUR MIND. "Do not conform any longer to the pattern of this world, but be transformed by the renewing of your mind" (Romans 12:2). Scripture memory allows you to replace a lie with the truth of God's Word. When Scripture becomes firmly settled in your memory, not only will your thoughts connect with God's thoughts, but you will also be able to honor God with small everyday decisions as well as big life-impacting ones. Scripture memorization is the key to making a permanent lifestyle change in your thought patterns, which brings balance to every other area of your life.

Scripture Memory Tips

- Write the verse down, saying it aloud as you write it.
- Read verses before and after the memory verse to get its context.
- Read the verse several times, emphasizing a different word each time.
- Connect the Scripture reference to the first few words.
- Locate patterns, phrases, or keywords.
- Apply the Scripture to circumstances you are now experiencing.
- Pray the verse, making it personal to your life and inserting your name as the recipient of the promise or teaching. (Try that with 1 Corinthians 10:13, inserting "me" and "I" for "you.")
- Review the verse every day until it becomes second nature to think those words whenever your circumstances match its message. The Holy Spirit will bring the verse to mind when you need it most if you decide to plant it in your memory.

Scripture Memorization Made Easy!

What is your learning style? Do you learn by hearing, by sight, or by doing? If you learn by hearing—if you are an auditory learner—singing the Scripture memory verses, reading them aloud, or recording them and listening to your recording will be very helpful in the memorization process. If you are a visual learner, writing the verses and repeatedly reading through them will cement them in your mind.

If you learn by doing—if you are a tactile learner—creating motions for the words or using sign language will enable you to more easily recall the verse. After determining your learning style, link your Scripture memory with a daily task, such as driving to work, walking on a treadmill, or eating lunch. Use these daily tasks as opportunities to memorize and review your verses.

Meals at home or out with friends can be used as a time to share the verse you are memorizing with those at your table. You could close your personal email messages by typing in your weekly memory verse. Or why not say your memory verse every time you brush your teeth or put on your shoes?

The purpose of Scripture memorization is to be able to apply God's words to your life. If you memorize Scripture using methods that connect with your particular learning style, you will find it easier to hide God's Word in your heart.

—— ESTABLISHING A QUIET TIME

Like all other components of the First Place for Health program, developing a live relationship with God is not a random act. You must intentionally seek God if you are to find Him! It's not that God plays hide-and-seek with you. He is always available to you. He invites you to come boldly into His presence. He reveals Himself to you in the pages of the Bible. And once you decide to earnestly seek Him, you are sure to find Him! When you delight in Him, your gracious God will give you the desires of your heart. Spending time getting to know God involves four basic elements: a priority, a plan, a place, and practice.

A Priority

You can successfully establish a quiet time with God by making this meeting a daily priority. This may require carving out time in your day so you have time and space for this new relationship you are cultivating. Often this will mean eliminating less important things so you will have time and space to meet with God. When speaking about Jesus, John the Baptist said, "He must become greater; I must become less" (John 3:30). You will undoubtedly find that to be true as well. What might you need to eliminate from your current schedule so that spending quality time with God can become a priority?

A Plan

Having made quiet time a priority, you will want to come up with a plan. This plan will include the time you have set aside to spend with God and a general outline of how you will spend your time in God's presence.

Elements you should consider incorporating into your quiet time include:

- Singing a song of praise
- Reading a daily selection in a devotional book or reading a psalm
- Using a systematic Scripture reading plan so you will be exposed to the whole truth of God's Word
- Completing your First Place for Health Bible study for that day
- Praying—silent, spoken, and written prayer
- Writing in your spiritual journal.

You will also want to make a list of the materials you will need to make your encounter with God more meaningful:

- A Bible
- Your First Place for Health Bible study
- Your prayer journal
- A pen and/or pencil
- A devotional book
- A Bible concordance
- A college-level dictionary
- A box of tissues (tears—both of sadness and joy—are often part of our quiet time with God!)

Think of how you would plan an important business meeting or social event, and then transfer that knowledge to your meeting time with God.

A Place

Having formulated a meeting-with-God plan, you will next need to create a meeting-with-God place. Of course, God is always with you; however, in order to have quality devotional time with Him, it is desirable that you find a comfortable meeting place. You will want to select a spot that is quiet and as distraction-free as possible.

Meeting with God in the same place on a regular basis will help you remember what you are there for: to have an encounter with the true and living God!

Having selected the place, put the materials you have determined to use in your quiet time into a basket or on a nearby table or shelf. Now take the time to establish your personal quiet time with God. Tailor your quiet time to fit your needs—and the time you have allotted to spend with God. Although many people elect to meet with God early in the morning, for others afternoon or evening is best. There is no hard-and-fast rule about when your quiet time should be—the only essential thing is that you establish a quiet time!

Start with a small amount of time that you know you can devote yourself to daily. You can be confident that as you consistently spend time with God each day, the amount of time you can spend will increase as you are ready for the next level of your walk with God.

I will meet with God from _____ to _____ daily.

I plan to use that time with God to _____

_____

Supplies I will need to assemble include _____

_____

My meeting place with God will be _____

_____

Practice

After you have chosen the time and place to meet God each day and you have assembled your supplies, there are four easy steps for having a fruitful and worshipful time with the Lord.

STEP 1: Clear Your Heart and Mind

"Be still, and know that I am God" (Psalm 46:10). Begin your quiet time by reading the daily Bible selection from a devotional guide or a psalm. If you are new in your Christian walk, an excellent devotional guide to use is *Streams in the Desert* by L.B. Cowman. More mature Christians might benefit from My Utmost for His Highest by Oswald Chambers. Of course, you can use any devotional that has a strong emphasis on Scripture and prayer.

STEP 2: Read and Interact with Scripture

"I have hidden your word in my heart that I might not sin against you" (Psalm 119:11). As you open your Bible, ask the Holy Spirit to reveal something He knows you need for this day through the reading of His Word. Always try to find a nugget to encourage or direct you through the day. As you read the passage, pay special attention to the words and phrases the Holy Spirit brings to your attention. Some words may seem to resonate in your soul. You will want to spend time meditating on the passage, asking God what lesson He is teaching you.

After reading the Scripture passage over several times, ask yourself the following questions:

- In light of what I have read today, is there something I must now do? (Confess a sin? Claim a promise? Follow an example? Obey a command? Avoid a situation?)
- How should I respond to what I've read today?

STEP 3: Pray

"Be clear minded and self-controlled so that you can pray" (1 Peter 4:7). Spend time conversing with the Lord in prayer. Prayer is such an important part of First Place for Health that there is an entire section in this member's guide devoted to the practice of prayer.

STEP 4: Praise

"Praise the LORD, O my soul, and forget not all his benefits" (Psalm 103:2). End your quiet time with a time of praise. Be sure to thank the Lord of heaven and warmth for choosing to spend time with you!

— SHARING YOUR FAITH

Nothing is more effective in drawing someone to Jesus than sharing personal life experiences. People are more open to the good news of Jesus Christ when they see faith in action. Personal faith stories are simple and effective ways to share what Christ is doing in your life, because they show firsthand how Christ makes a difference.

Sharing your faith story has an added benefit: it builds you up in your faith, too! Is your experience in First Place for Health providing you opportunities to share with others what God is doing in your life? If you answered yes, then you have a personal faith story! If you do not have a personal faith story, perhaps it is because you don't know Jesus Christ as your personal Lord and Savior. Read through "Steps to Becoming a Christian" (which is the next chapter) and begin today to give Christ first place in your life.

Creativity and preparation in using opportunities to share a word or story about Jesus is an important part of the Christian life. Is Jesus helping you in a special way? Are you achieving a level of success or peace that you haven't experienced in other attempts to lose weight, exercise regularly, or eat healthier? As people see you making changes and achieving success, they may ask you how you are doing it. How will—or do—you respond? Remember, your story is unique, and it may allow others to see what Christ is doing in your life. It may also help to bring Christ into the life of another person.

Personal Statements of Faith

First Place for Health gives you a great opportunity to communicate your faith and express what God is doing in your life. Be ready to use your own personal statement of faith whenever the opportunity presents itself. Personal statements of faith should be short and fit naturally into a conversation. They don't require or expect any action or response from the listener. The goal is not to get another person to change but simply to help you communicate who you are and what's important to you.

Here are some examples of short statements of faith that you might use when someone asks what you are doing to lose weight:

- "I've been meeting with a group at my church. We pray together, support each other, learn about nutrition, and study the Bible."

- "It's amazing how Bible study and prayer are helping me lose weight and eat healthier."
- "I've had a lot of support from a group I meet with at church."
- "I'm relying more on God to help me make changes in my lifestyle."

Begin keeping a list of your meaningful experiences as you go through the First Place for Health program. Also notice what is happening in the lives of others. Use the following questions to help you prepare short personal statements and stories of faith:

- What is God doing in your life physically, mentally, emotionally, and spiritually?
- How has your relationship with God changed? Is it more intimate or personal?
- How is prayer, Bible study, and/or the support of others helping you achieve your goals for a healthy weight and good nutrition?

Writing Your Personal Faith Story

Write a brief story about how God is working in your life through First Place for Health. Use your story to help you share with others what's happening in your life.

Use the following questions to help develop your story:

- Why did you join First Place for Health? What specific circumstances led you to a Christ-centered health and weight-loss program? What were you feeling when you joined?
- What was your relationship with Christ when you started First Place for Health? What is it now?
- Has your experience in First Place for Health changed your relationship with Christ? With yourself? With others?
- How has your relationship with Christ, prayer, Bible study, and group support made a difference in your life?
- What specific verse or passage of Scripture has made a difference in the way you view yourself or your relationship with Christ?
- What experiences have impacted your life since starting First Place for Health?
- In what ways is Christ working in your life today? In what ways is He meeting your needs?

- How has Christ worked in other members of your First Place for Health group?

Answer the above questions in a few sentences, and then use your answers to help you write your own short personal faith story.

MEMBER SURVEY

We would love to know more about you. Share this form with your leader.

Name _____   Birth date _____

Tell us about your family.

_____

_____

_____

_____

Would you like to receive more information   Yes   No
about our church?

What area of expertise would you be willing to share with our class?

_____

_____

Why did you join First Place for Health?

_____

_____

With notice, would you be willing to lead a Bible study   Yes   No
discussion one week?

Are you comfortable praying out loud?   _____

Would you be willing to assist recording weights and/or   Yes   No
evaluating the Live It Trackers?

Any other comments:

_____

_____

PERSONAL WEIGHT AND MEASUREMENT RECORD

WEEK	WEIGHT	+ OR -	GOAL THIS SESSION	POUNDS TO GOAL
1				
2				
3				
4				
5				
6				
7				
8				
9				
10				
11				
12				

BEGINNING MEASUREMENTS

WAIST _____   HIPS _____   THIGHS _____   CHEST _____

ENDING MEASUREMENTS

WAIST _____   HIPS _____   THIGHS _____   CHEST _____

All athletes are disciplined in their training. They do it to win a prize that will fade away, but we do it for an eternal prize. 1 Corinthians 9:25

Date: _____

Name: _____

Home Phone: _____

Cell Phone: _____

Email: _____

Personal Prayer Concerns

_____

_____

_____

_____

_____

_____

_____

This form is for prayer requests that are personal to you and your journey in First Place for Health. Please complete and have it ready to turn in when you arrive at your group meeting.

Therefore, since we are surrounded by such a huge crowd of witnesses to the life of faith, let us strip off every weight that slows us down, especially the sin that so easily trips us up. And let us run with endurance the race God has set before us.
Hebrews 12:1

Date: _____

Name: _____

Home Phone: _____

Cell Phone: _____

Email: _____

Personal Prayer Concerns

_____

_____

_____

_____

_____

_____

_____

_____

This form is for prayer requests that are personal to you and your journey in First Place for Health. Please complete and have it ready to turn in when you arrive at your group meeting.

We do this by keeping our eyes on Jesus, the champion who initiates
and perfects our faith. Hebrews 12:2

Date: _____

Name: _____

Home Phone: _____

Cell Phone: _____

Email: _____

Personal Prayer Concerns

_____

_____

_____

_____

_____

_____

_____

_____

This form is for prayer requests that are personal to you and your journey in First Place for Health.
Please complete and have it ready to turn in when you arrive at your group meeting.

Commit everything you do to the Lord. Trust Him, and he will help
you. Psalm 37:5

Date: _____

Name: _____

Home Phone: _____

Cell Phone: _____

Email: _____

Personal Prayer Concerns

_____

_____

_____

_____

_____

_____

_____

_____

This form is for prayer requests that are personal to you and your journey in First Place for Health. Please complete and have it ready to turn in when you arrive at your group meeting.

So take a new grip with your tired hands and strengthen your weak knees. Mark out a straight path for your feet so that those who are weak and lame will not fall but become strong. Hebrews 12:12-13

Date: _____

Name: _____

Home Phone: _____

Cell Phone: _____

Email: _____

Personal Prayer Concerns

_____

_____

_____

_____

_____

_____

_____

_____

This form is for prayer requests that are personal to you and your journey in First Place for Health. Please complete and have it ready to turn in when you arrive at your group meeting.

No discipline is enjoyable while it is happening—it's painful! But afterward there will be a peaceful harvest of right living for those who are trained in this way. Hebrews 12:11

Date: _____

Name: _____

Home Phone: _____

Cell Phone: _____

Email: _____

Personal Prayer Concerns

_____

_____

_____

_____

_____

_____

_____

_____

This form is for prayer requests that are personal to you and your journey in First Place for Health. Please complete and have it ready to turn in when you arrive at your group meeting.

The temptations in your life are no different from what others experience. And God is faithful. He will not allow the temptation to be more than you can stand. When you are tempted, He will show you a way out so that you can endure. 1 Corinthians 10:13

Date: _____

Name: _____

Home Phone: _____

Cell Phone: _____

Email: _____

Personal Prayer Concerns

_____

_____

_____

_____

_____

_____

_____

_____

This form is for prayer requests that are personal to you and your journey in First Place for Health. Please complete and have it ready to turn in when you arrive at your group meeting.

The God of peace will soon crush Satan under your feet. May the grace of our Lord
Jesus be with you. Romans 16:20

Date: ....

Name: ....

Home Phone: ....

Cell Phone: ....

Email: ....

Personal Prayer Concern

This form is for prayer requests that are personal to you and your journey in First Place for Health.
Please complete and have it ready to turn in when you arrive at your group meeting.

PRAYER PARTNER

Date: _____

Name: _____

Home Phone: _____

Cell Phone: _____

Email: _____

Personal Prayer Concerns

_____

_____

_____

_____

_____

_____

_____

This form is for prayer requests that are personal to you and your journey in First Place for Health. Please complete and have it ready to turn in when you arrive at your group meeting.

LIVE IT TRACKER

Name: _____

Date: _____ Week #: _____

My activity goal for next week:
○ None   ○ <30 min/day   ○ 30-60 min/day

My food goal for next week: _____
_____

loss/gain _____   Calorie Range: _____

My week at a glance:
○ Great   ○ So-so   ○ Not so great

Activity level:
○ None   ○ <30 min/day   ○ 30-60 min/day

RECOMMENDED DAILY AMOUNT OF FOOD FROM EACH GROUP

GROUP	DAILY CALORIES							
	1300-1400	1500-1600	1700-1800	1900-2000	2100-2200	2300-2400	2500-2600	2700-2800
Fruits	1.5 – 2 c.	1.5 – 2 c.	1.5 – 2 c.	2 - 2.5 c.	2 – 2.5 c.	2.5 – 3.5 c.	3.5 – 4.5 c.	3.5 – 4.5 c.
Vegetables	1.5 – 2 c.	2 - 2.5 c.	2.5 – 3 c.	2.5 – 3 c.	3 – 3.5 c.	3.5 – 4.5 c.	4.5 – 5 c.	4.5 – 5 c.
Grains	5 oz eq.	5-6 oz eq.	6-7 oz eq.	6-7 oz eq.	7-8 oz eq.	8-9 oz eq.	9-10 oz eq.	10-11 oz eq.
Dairy	2-3 c.	3 c.	3 c.	3 c.	3 c.	3 c.	3 c.	3 c.
Protein	4 oz eq.	5 oz eq.	5-5.5 oz eq.	5.5-6.5 oz eq.	6.5-7 oz eq.	7-7.5 oz eq.	7-7.5 oz eq.	7.5-8 oz eq.
Healthy Oils & Other Fats	4 tsp.	5 tsp.	5 tsp.	6 tsp.	6 tsp.	7 tsp.	8 tsp.	8 tsp.
Water & Super Beverages*	Women: 9 c. Men: 13 c.	Women: 9 c. Men: 13 c.	Women: 9 c. Men: 13 c.	Women: 9 c. Men: 13 c.	Women: 9 c. Men: 13 c.	Women: 9 c. Men: 13 c.	Women: 9 c. Men: 13 c.	Women: 9 c. Men: 13 c.

*May count up to 3 cups caffeinated tea or coffee toward goal

DAILY FOOD GROUP TRACKER

GROUP	FRUITS	VEGETABLES	GRAINS	PROTEIN	DAIRY	HEALTHY OILS & OTHER FATS	WATER & SUPER BEVERAGES
1 Estimate Total							
2 Estimate Total							
3 Estimate Total							
4 Estimate Total							
5 Estimate Total							
6 Estimate Total							
7 Estimate Total							

FOOD CHOICES   DAY ❶

Breakfast: _____
Lunch: _____
Dinner: _____
Snacks: _____

PHYSICAL ACTIVITY   steps/miles/minutes: _____

description: _____

SPIRITUAL ACTIVITY

description: _____

FOOD CHOICES — DAY ❷

Breakfast: _____
Lunch: _____
Dinner: _____
Snacks: _____

PHYSICAL ACTIVITY — steps/miles/minutes:
description: _____
_____

SPIRITUAL ACTIVITY
description: _____

FOOD CHOICES — DAY ❸

Breakfast: _____
Lunch: _____
Dinner: _____
Snacks: _____

PHYSICAL ACTIVITY — steps/miles/minutes:
description: _____
_____

SPIRITUAL ACTIVITY
description: _____

FOOD CHOICES — DAY ❹

Breakfast: _____
Lunch: _____
Dinner: _____
Snacks: _____

PHYSICAL ACTIVITY — steps/miles/minutes:
description: _____
_____

SPIRITUAL ACTIVITY
description: _____

FOOD CHOICES — DAY ❺

Breakfast: _____
Lunch: _____
Dinner: _____
Snacks: _____

PHYSICAL ACTIVITY — steps/miles/minutes:
description: _____
_____

SPIRITUAL ACTIVITY
description: _____

FOOD CHOICES — DAY ❻

Breakfast: _____
Lunch: _____
Dinner: _____
Snacks: _____

PHYSICAL ACTIVITY — steps/miles/minutes:
description: _____
_____

SPIRITUAL ACTIVITY
description: _____

FOOD CHOICES — DAY ❼

Breakfast: _____
Lunch: _____
Dinner: _____
Snacks: _____

PHYSICAL ACTIVITY — steps/miles/minutes:
description: _____
_____

SPIRITUAL ACTIVITY
description: _____

LIVE IT TRACKER

Name: _____

Date: _____ Week #: _____

My activity goal for next week:
○ None   ○ <30 min/day   ○ 30-60 min/day

loss/gain _____ Calorie Range: _____

My week at a glance:
○ Great   ○ So-so   ○ Not so great

Activity level:
○ None   ○ <30 min/day   ○ 30-60 min/day

My food goal for next week: _____
_____

RECOMMENDED DAILY AMOUNT OF FOOD FROM EACH GROUP

GROUP	DAILY CALORIES							
	1300-1400	1500-1600	1700-1800	1900-2000	2100-2200	2300-2400	2500-2600	2700-2800
Fruits	1.5 – 2 c.	1.5 – 2 c.	1.5 – 2 c.	2 – 2.5 c.	2 – 2.5 c.	2.5 – 3.5 c.	3.5 – 4.5 c.	3.5 – 4.5 c.
Vegetables	1.5 – 2 c.	2 – 2.5 c.	2.5 – 3 c.	2.5 – 3 c.	3 – 3.5 c.	3.5 – 4.5 c.	4.5 – 5 c.	4.5 – 5 c.
Grains	5 oz eq.	5-6 oz eq.	6-7 oz eq.	6-7 oz eq.	7-8 oz eq.	8-9 oz eq.	9-10 oz eq.	10-11 oz eq.
Dairy	2-3 c.	3 c.	3 c.	3 c.	3 c.	3 c.	3 c.	3 c.
Protein	4 oz eq.	5 oz eq.	5-5.5 oz eq.	5.5-6.5 oz eq.	6.5-7 oz eq.	7-7.5 oz eq.	7-7.5 oz eq.	7.5-8 oz eq.
Healthy Oils & Other Fats	4 tsp.	5 tsp.	5 tsp.	6 tsp.	6 tsp.	7 tsp.	8 tsp.	8 tsp.
Water & Super Beverages*	Women: 9 c. Men: 13 c.	Women: 9 c. Men: 13 c.	Women: 9 c. Men: 13 c.	Women: 9 c. Men: 13 c.	Women: 9 c. Men: 13 c.	Women: 9 c. Men: 13 c.	Women: 9 c. Men: 13 c.	Women: 9 c. Men: 13 c.

*May count up to 3 cups caffeinated tea or coffee toward goal

DAILY FOOD GROUP TRACKER

GROUP	FRUITS	VEGETABLES	GRAINS	PROTEIN	DAIRY	HEALTHY OILS & OTHER FATS	WATER & SUPER BEVERAGES
1 Estimate Total							
2 Estimate Total							
3 Estimate Total							
4 Estimate Total							
5 Estimate Total							
6 Estimate Total							
7 Estimate Total							

FOOD CHOICES   DAY 1

Breakfast: _____
Lunch: _____
Dinner: _____
Snacks: _____

PHYSICAL ACTIVITY   steps/miles/minutes: _____

description: _____

SPIRITUAL ACTIVITY

description: _____

FOOD CHOICES

DAY 2

Breakfast: _____
Lunch: _____
Dinner: _____
Snacks: _____

PHYSICAL ACTIVITY steps/miles/minutes:

description: _____

SPIRITUAL ACTIVITY

description: _____

FOOD CHOICES

DAY 3

Breakfast: _____
Lunch: _____
Dinner: _____
Snacks: _____

PHYSICAL ACTIVITY steps/miles/minutes:

description: _____

SPIRITUAL ACTIVITY

description: _____

FOOD CHOICES

DAY 4

Breakfast: _____
Lunch: _____
Dinner: _____
Snacks: _____

PHYSICAL ACTIVITY steps/miles/minutes:

description: _____

SPIRITUAL ACTIVITY

description: _____

FOOD CHOICES

DAY 5

Breakfast: _____
Lunch: _____
Dinner: _____
Snacks: _____

PHYSICAL ACTIVITY steps/miles/minutes:

description: _____

SPIRITUAL ACTIVITY

description: _____

FOOD CHOICES

DAY 6

Breakfast: _____
Lunch: _____
Dinner: _____
Snacks: _____

PHYSICAL ACTIVITY steps/miles/minutes:

description: _____

SPIRITUAL ACTIVITY

description: _____

FOOD CHOICES

DAY 7

Breakfast: _____
Lunch: _____
Dinner: _____
Snacks: _____

PHYSICAL ACTIVITY steps/miles/minutes:

description: _____

SPIRITUAL ACTIVITY

description: _____

LIVE IT TRACKER

Name: _____

Date: _____ Week #: _____

My activity goal for next week:
○ None ○ <30 min/day ○ 30-60 min/day

loss/gain _____ Calorie Range: _____

My week at a glance:
○ Great ○ So-so ○ Not so great

My food goal for next week: _____

Activity level:
○ None ○ <30 min/day ○ 30-60 min/day

RECOMMENDED DAILY AMOUNT OF FOOD FROM EACH GROUP

GROUP	DAILY CALORIES							
....	1300-1400	1500-1600	1700-1800	1900-2000	2100-2200	2300-2400	2500-2600	2700-2800
Fruits	1.5 – 2 c.	1.5 – 2 c.	1.5 – 2 c.	2 – 2.5 c.	2 – 2.5 c.	2.5 – 3.5 c.	3.5 – 4.5 c.	3.5 – 4.5 c.
Vegetables	1.5 – 2 c.	2 – 2.5 c.	2.5 – 3 c.	2.5 – 3 c.	3 – 3.5 c.	3.5 – 4.5 c.	4.5 – 5 c.	4.5 – 5 c.
Grains	5 oz eq.	5-6 oz eq.	6-7 oz eq.	6-7 oz eq.	7-8 oz eq.	8-9 oz eq.	9-10 oz eq.	10-11 oz eq.
Dairy	2-3 c.	3 c.	3 c.	3 c.	3 c.	3 c.	3 c.	3 c.
Protein	4 oz eq.	5 oz eq.	5-5.5 oz eq.	5.5-6.5 oz eq.	6.5-7 oz eq.	7-7.5 oz eq.	7-7.5 oz eq.	7.5-8 oz eq.
Healthy Oils & Other Fats	4 tsp.	5 tsp.	5 tsp.	6 tsp.	6 tsp.	7 tsp.	8 tsp.	8 tsp.
Water & Super Beverages*	Women: 9 c. Men: 13 c.	Women: 9 c. Men: 13 c.	Women: 9 c. Men: 13 c.	Women: 9 c. Men: 13 c.	Women: 9 c. Men: 13 c.	Women: 9 c. Men: 13 c.	Women: 9 c. Men: 13 c.	Women: 9 c. Men: 13 c.

*May count up to 3 cups caffeinated tea or coffee toward goal

DAILY FOOD GROUP TRACKER

	GROUP	FRUITS	VEGETABLES	GRAINS	PROTEIN	DAIRY	HEALTHY OILS & OTHER FATS	WATER & SUPER BEVERAGES
1	Estimate Total							
2	Estimate Total							
3	Estimate Total							
4	Estimate Total							
5	Estimate Total							
6	Estimate Total							
7	Estimate Total							

FOOD CHOICES

DAY 1

Breakfast: _____
Lunch: _____
Dinner: _____
Snacks: _____

PHYSICAL ACTIVITY steps/miles/minutes: _____

description: _____

SPIRITUAL ACTIVITY

description: _____

FOOD CHOICES   DAY ❷

Breakfast: _____
Lunch: _____
Dinner: _____
Snacks: _____

PHYSICAL ACTIVITY   steps/miles/minutes: _____   SPIRITUAL ACTIVITY

description: _____   description: _____
_____   _____

FOOD CHOICES   DAY ❸

Breakfast: _____
Lunch: _____
Dinner: _____
Snacks: _____

PHYSICAL ACTIVITY   steps/miles/minutes: _____   SPIRITUAL ACTIVITY

description: _____   description: _____
_____   _____

FOOD CHOICES   DAY ❹

Breakfast: _____
Lunch: _____
Dinner: _____
Snacks: _____

PHYSICAL ACTIVITY   steps/miles/minutes: _____   SPIRITUAL ACTIVITY

description: _____   description: _____
_____   _____

FOOD CHOICES   DAY ❺

Breakfast: _____
Lunch: _____
Dinner: _____
Snacks: _____

PHYSICAL ACTIVITY   steps/miles/minutes: _____   SPIRITUAL ACTIVITY

description: _____   description: _____
_____   _____

FOOD CHOICES   DAY ❻

Breakfast: _____
Lunch: _____
Dinner: _____
Snacks: _____

PHYSICAL ACTIVITY   steps/miles/minutes: _____   SPIRITUAL ACTIVITY

description: _____   description: _____
_____   _____

FOOD CHOICES   DAY ❼

Breakfast: _____
Lunch: _____
Dinner: _____
Snacks: _____

PHYSICAL ACTIVITY   steps/miles/minutes: _____   SPIRITUAL ACTIVITY

description: _____   description: _____
_____   _____

LIVE IT TRACKER

Name: _____

My activity goal for next week:
○ None   ○ <30 min/day   ○ 30-60 min/day

My food goal for next week: _____
_____

Date: _____ Week #: _____

loss/gain _____ Calorie Range: _____

My week at a glance:
○ Great   ○ So-so   ○ Not so great

Activity level:
○ None   ○ <30 min/day   ○ 30-60 min/day

RECOMMENDED DAILY AMOUNT OF FOOD FROM EACH GROUP

GROUP	DAILY CALORIES							
	1300-1400	1500-1600	1700-1800	1900-2000	2100-2200	2300-2400	2500-2600	2700-2800
Fruits	1.5 – 2 c.	1.5 – 2 c.	1.5 – 2 c.	2 – 2.5 c.	2 – 2.5 c.	2.5 – 3.5 c.	3.5 – 4.5 c.	3.5 – 4.5 c.
Vegetables	1.5 – 2 c.	2 – 2.5 c.	2.5 – 3 c.	2.5 – 3 c.	3 – 3.5 c.	3.5 – 4.5 c.	4.5 – 5 c.	4.5 – 5 c.
Grains	5 oz eq.	5-6 oz eq.	6-7 oz eq.	6-7 oz eq.	7-8 oz eq.	8-9 oz eq.	9-10 oz eq.	10-11 oz eq.
Dairy	2-3 c.	3 c.	3 c.	3 c.	3 c.	3 c.	3 c.	3 c.
Protein	4 oz eq.	5 oz eq.	5-5.5 oz eq.	5.5-6.5 oz eq.	6.5-7 oz eq.	7-7.5 oz eq.	7-7.5 oz eq.	7.5-8 oz eq.
Healthy Oils & Other Fats	4 tsp.	5 tsp.	5 tsp.	6 tsp.	6 tsp.	7 tsp.	8 tsp.	8 tsp.
Water & Super Beverages*	Women: 9 c. Men: 13 c.	Women: 9 c. Men: 13 c.	Women: 9 c. Men: 13 c.	Women: 9 c. Men: 13 c.	Women: 9 c. Men: 13 c.	Women: 9 c. Men: 13 c.	Women: 9 c. Men: 13 c.	Women: 9 c. Men: 13 c.

*May count up to 3 cups caffeinated tea or coffee toward goal

DAILY FOOD GROUP TRACKER

	GROUP	FRUITS	VEGETABLES	GRAINS	PROTEIN	DAIRY	HEALTHY OILS & OTHER FATS	WATER & SUPER BEVERAGES
1	Estimate Total							
2	Estimate Total							
3	Estimate Total							
4	Estimate Total							
5	Estimate Total							
6	Estimate Total							
7	Estimate Total							

FOOD CHOICES   DAY ❶

Breakfast: _____
Lunch: _____
Dinner: _____
Snacks: _____

PHYSICAL ACTIVITY   steps/miles/minutes: _____

description: _____
_____

SPIRITUAL ACTIVITY

description: _____

FOOD CHOICES — DAY 2

Breakfast: _____
Lunch: _____
Dinner: _____
Snacks: _____

PHYSICAL ACTIVITY   steps/miles/minutes: _____

description: _____
_____

SPIRITUAL ACTIVITY

description: _____
_____

FOOD CHOICES — DAY 3

Breakfast: _____
Lunch: _____
Dinner: _____
Snacks: _____

PHYSICAL ACTIVITY   steps/miles/minutes: _____

description: _____
_____

SPIRITUAL ACTIVITY

description: _____
_____

FOOD CHOICES — DAY 4

Breakfast: _____
Lunch: _____
Dinner: _____
Snacks: _____

PHYSICAL ACTIVITY   steps/miles/minutes: _____

description: _____
_____

SPIRITUAL ACTIVITY

description: _____
_____

FOOD CHOICES — DAY 5

Breakfast: _____
Lunch: _____
Dinner: _____
Snacks: _____

PHYSICAL ACTIVITY   steps/miles/minutes: _____

description: _____
_____

SPIRITUAL ACTIVITY

description: _____
_____

FOOD CHOICES — DAY 6

Breakfast: _____
Lunch: _____
Dinner: _____
Snacks: _____

PHYSICAL ACTIVITY   steps/miles/minutes: _____

description: _____
_____

SPIRITUAL ACTIVITY

description: _____
_____

FOOD CHOICES — DAY 7

Breakfast: _____
Lunch: _____
Dinner: _____
Snacks: _____

PHYSICAL ACTIVITY   steps/miles/minutes: _____

description: _____
_____

SPIRITUAL ACTIVITY

description: _____
_____

LIVE IT TRACKER

Name: _____

Date: _____ Week #: _____

My activity goal for next week:
○ None   ○ <30 min/day   ○ 30-60 min/day

My food goal for next week: _____
_____

loss/gain _____ Calorie Range: _____

My week at a glance:
○ Great   ○ So-so   ○ Not so great

Activity level:
○ None   ○ <30 min/day   ○ 30-60 min/day

RECOMMENDED DAILY AMOUNT OF FOOD FROM EACH GROUP

GROUP	DAILY CALORIES							
....	1300-1400	1500-1600	1700-1800	1900-2000	2100-2200	2300-2400	2500-2600	2700-2800
Fruits	1.5 – 2 c.	1.5 – 2 c.	1.5 – 2 c.	2 – 2.5 c.	2 – 2.5 c.	2.5 – 3.5 c.	3.5 – 4.5 c.	3.5 – 4.5 c.
Vegetables	1.5 – 2 c.	2 – 2.5 c.	2.5 – 3 c.	2.5 – 3 c.	3 – 3.5 c.	3.5 – 4.5 c.	4.5 – 5 c.	4.5 – 5 c.
Grains	5 oz eq.	5-6 oz eq.	6-7 oz eq.	6-7 oz eq.	7-8 oz eq.	8-9 oz eq.	9-10 oz eq.	10-11 oz eq.
Dairy	2-3 c.	3 c.	3 c.	3 c.	3 c.	3 c.	3 c.	3 c.
Protein	4 oz eq.	5 oz eq.	5-5.5 oz eq.	5.5-6.5 oz eq.	6.5-7 oz eq.	7-7.5 oz eq.	7-7.5 oz eq.	7.5-8 oz eq.
Healthy Oils & Other Fats	4 tsp.	5 tsp.	5 tsp.	6 tsp.	6 tsp.	7 tsp.	8 tsp.	8 tsp.
Water & Super Beverages*	Women: 9 c. Men: 13 c.	Women: 9 c. Men: 13 c.	Women: 9 c. Men: 13 c.	Women: 9 c. Men: 13 c.	Women: 9 c. Men: 13 c.	Women: 9 c. Men: 13 c.	Women: 9 c. Men: 13 c.	Women: 9 c. Men: 13 c.

*May count up to 3 cups caffeinated tea or coffee toward goal

DAILY FOOD GROUP TRACKER

GROUP	FRUITS	VEGETABLES	GRAINS	PROTEIN	DAIRY	HEALTHY OILS & OTHER FATS	WATER & SUPER BEVERAGES
❶ Estimate Total							
❷ Estimate Total							
❸ Estimate Total							
❹ Estimate Total							
❺ Estimate Total							
❻ Estimate Total							
❼ Estimate Total							

FOOD CHOICES   DAY ❶

Breakfast: _____
Lunch: _____
Dinner: _____
Snacks: _____

PHYSICAL ACTIVITY   steps/miles/minutes: _____

description: _____

SPIRITUAL ACTIVITY

description: _____

FOOD CHOICES

DAY ❷

Breakfast: _____
Lunch: _____
Dinner: _____
Snacks: _____

PHYSICAL ACTIVITY steps/miles/minutes: _____

description: _____
_____

SPIRITUAL ACTIVITY

description: _____
_____

FOOD CHOICES

DAY ❸

Breakfast: _____
Lunch: _____
Dinner: _____
Snacks: _____

PHYSICAL ACTIVITY steps/miles/minutes: _____

description: _____
_____

SPIRITUAL ACTIVITY

description: _____
_____

FOOD CHOICES

DAY ❹

Breakfast: _____
Lunch: _____
Dinner: _____
Snacks: _____

PHYSICAL ACTIVITY steps/miles/minutes: _____

description: _____
_____

SPIRITUAL ACTIVITY

description: _____
_____

FOOD CHOICES

DAY ❺

Breakfast: _____
Lunch: _____
Dinner: _____
Snacks: _____

PHYSICAL ACTIVITY steps/miles/minutes: _____

description: _____
_____

SPIRITUAL ACTIVITY

description: _____
_____

FOOD CHOICES

DAY ❻

Breakfast: _____
Lunch: _____
Dinner: _____
Snacks: _____

PHYSICAL ACTIVITY steps/miles/minutes: _____

description: _____
_____

SPIRITUAL ACTIVITY

description: _____
_____

FOOD CHOICES

DAY ❼

Breakfast: _____
Lunch: _____
Dinner: _____
Snacks: _____

PHYSICAL ACTIVITY steps/miles/minutes: _____

description: _____
_____

SPIRITUAL ACTIVITY

description: _____
_____

LIVE IT TRACKER

Name: _____

Date: _____ Week #: _____

My activity goal for next week:
- ○ None   ○ <30 min/day   ○ 30-60 min/day

loss/gain _____   Calorie Range: _____

My food goal for next week: _____

My week at a glance:
- ○ Great   ○ So-so   ○ Not so great

Activity level:
- ○ None   ○ <30 min/day   ○ 30-60 min/day

RECOMMENDED DAILY AMOUNT OF FOOD FROM EACH GROUP

GROUP	DAILY CALORIES							
....	1300-1400	1500-1600	1700-1800	1900-2000	2100-2200	2300-2400	2500-2600	2700-2800
Fruits	1.5 – 2 c.	1.5 – 2 c.	1.5 – 2 c.	2 – 2.5 c.	2 – 2.5 c.	2.5 – 3.5 c.	3.5 – 4.5 c.	3.5 – 4.5 c.
Vegetables	1.5 – 2 c.	2 – 2.5 c.	2.5 – 3 c.	2.5 – 3 c.	3 – 3.5 c.	3.5 – 4.5 c.	4.5 – 5 c.	4.5 – 5 c.
Grains	5 oz eq.	5-6 oz eq.	6-7 oz eq.	6-7 oz eq.	7-8 oz eq.	8-9 oz eq.	9-10 oz eq.	10-11 oz eq.
Dairy	2-3 c.	3 c.	3 c.	3 c.	3 c.	3 c.	3 c.	3 c.
Protein	4 oz eq.	5 oz eq.	5-5.5 oz eq.	5.5-6.5 oz eq.	6.5-7 oz eq.	7-7.5 oz eq.	7-7.5 oz eq.	7.5-8 oz eq.
Healthy Oils & Other Fats	4 tsp.	5 tsp.	5 tsp.	6 tsp.	6 tsp.	7 tsp.	8 tsp.	8 tsp.
Water & Super Beverages*	Women: 9 c. Men: 13 c.	Women: 9 c. Men: 13 c.	Women: 9 c. Men: 13 c.	Women: 9 c. Men: 13 c.	Women: 9 c. Men: 13 c.	Women: 9 c. Men: 13 c.	Women: 9 c. Men: 13 c.	Women: 9 c. Men: 13 c.

*May count up to 3 cups caffeinated tea or coffee toward goal

DAILY FOOD GROUP TRACKER

GROUP	FRUITS	VEGETABLES	GRAINS	PROTEIN	DAIRY	HEALTHY OILS & OTHER FATS	WATER & SUPER BEVERAGES
1 Estimate Total							
2 Estimate Total							
3 Estimate Total							
4 Estimate Total							
5 Estimate Total							
6 Estimate Total							
7 Estimate Total							

FOOD CHOICES   DAY 1

Breakfast: _____
Lunch: _____
Dinner: _____
Snacks: _____

PHYSICAL ACTIVITY   steps/miles/minutes: _____

description: _____

SPIRITUAL ACTIVITY

description: _____

FOOD CHOICES   DAY ❷

Breakfast: _____

Lunch: _____

Dinner: _____

Snacks: _____

PHYSICAL ACTIVITY steps/miles/minutes:	SPIRITUAL ACTIVITY
description: _____	description: _____
_____	_____

FOOD CHOICES   DAY ❸

Breakfast: _____

Lunch: _____

Dinner: _____

Snacks: _____

PHYSICAL ACTIVITY steps/miles/minutes:	SPIRITUAL ACTIVITY
description: _____	description: _____
_____	_____

FOOD CHOICES   DAY ❹

Breakfast: _____

Lunch: _____

Dinner: _____

Snacks: _____

PHYSICAL ACTIVITY steps/miles/minutes:	SPIRITUAL ACTIVITY
description: _____	description: _____
_____	_____

FOOD CHOICES   DAY ❺

Breakfast: _____

Lunch: _____

Dinner: _____

Snacks: _____

PHYSICAL ACTIVITY steps/miles/minutes:	SPIRITUAL ACTIVITY
description: _____	description: _____
_____	_____

FOOD CHOICES   DAY ❻

Breakfast: _____

Lunch: _____

Dinner: _____

Snacks: _____

PHYSICAL ACTIVITY steps/miles/minutes:	SPIRITUAL ACTIVITY
description: _____	description: _____
_____	_____

FOOD CHOICES   DAY ❼

Breakfast: _____

Lunch: _____

Dinner: _____

Snacks: _____

PHYSICAL ACTIVITY steps/miles/minutes:	SPIRITUAL ACTIVITY
description: _____	description: _____
_____	_____

LIVE IT TRACKER

Name: _____

My activity goal for next week:
○ None   ○ <30 min/day   ○ 30-60 min/day

My food goal for next week: _____
_____

Date: _____ Week #: _____

loss/gain _____ Calorie Range: _____

My week at a glance:
○ Great   ○ So-so   ○ Not so great

Activity level:
○ None   ○ <30 min/day   ○ 30-60 min/day

RECOMMENDED DAILY AMOUNT OF FOOD FROM EACH GROUP

GROUP	DAILY CALORIES							
	1300-1400	1500-1600	1700-1800	1900-2000	2100-2200	2300-2400	2500-2600	2700-2800
Fruits	1.5 – 2 c.	1.5 – 2 c.	1.5 – 2 c.	2 – 2.5 c.	2 – 2.5 c.	2.5 – 3.5 c.	3.5 – 4.5 c.	3.5 – 4.5 c.
Vegetables	1.5 – 2 c.	2 – 2.5 c.	2.5 – 3 c.	2.5 – 3 c.	3 – 3.5 c.	3.5 – 4.5 c.	4.5 – 5 c.	4.5 – 5 c.
Grains	5 oz eq.	5-6 oz eq.	6-7 oz eq.	6-7 oz eq.	7-8 oz eq.	8-9 oz eq.	9-10 oz eq.	10-11 oz eq.
Dairy	2-3 c.	3 c.	3 c.	3 c.	3 c.	3 c.	3 c.	3 c.
Protein	4 oz eq.	5 oz eq.	5-5.5 oz eq.	5.5-6.5 oz eq.	6.5-7 oz eq.	7-7.5 oz eq.	7-7.5 oz eq.	7.5-8 oz eq.
Healthy Oils & Other Fats	4 tsp.	5 tsp.	5 tsp.	6 tsp.	6 tsp.	7 tsp.	8 tsp.	8 tsp.
Water & Super Beverages*	Women: 9 c. Men: 13 c.	Women: 9 c. Men: 13 c.	Women: 9 c. Men: 13 c.	Women: 9 c. Men: 13 c.	Women: 9 c. Men: 13 c.	Women: 9 c. Men: 13 c.	Women: 9 c. Men: 13 c.	Women: 9 c. Men: 13 c.

*May count up to 3 cups caffeinated tea or coffee toward goal

DAILY FOOD GROUP TRACKER

GROUP	FRUITS	VEGETABLES	GRAINS	PROTEIN	DAIRY	HEALTHY OILS & OTHER FATS	WATER & SUPER BEVERAGES
1 Estimate Total							
2 Estimate Total							
3 Estimate Total							
4 Estimate Total							
5 Estimate Total							
6 Estimate Total							
7 Estimate Total							

FOOD CHOICES   **DAY ❶**

Breakfast: _____
Lunch: _____
Dinner: _____
Snacks: _____

PHYSICAL ACTIVITY   steps/miles/minutes: _____

description: _____

SPIRITUAL ACTIVITY

description: _____

FOOD CHOICES DAY ❷

Breakfast: _____
Lunch: _____
Dinner: _____
Snacks: _____

PHYSICAL ACTIVITY steps/miles/minutes: _____

description: _____

SPIRITUAL ACTIVITY

description: _____

FOOD CHOICES DAY ❸

Breakfast: _____
Lunch: _____
Dinner: _____
Snacks: _____

PHYSICAL ACTIVITY steps/miles/minutes: _____

description: _____

SPIRITUAL ACTIVITY

description: _____

FOOD CHOICES DAY ❹

Breakfast: _____
Lunch: _____
Dinner: _____
Snacks: _____

PHYSICAL ACTIVITY steps/miles/minutes: _____

description: _____

SPIRITUAL ACTIVITY

description: _____

FOOD CHOICES DAY ❺

Breakfast: _____
Lunch: _____
Dinner: _____
Snacks: _____

PHYSICAL ACTIVITY steps/miles/minutes: _____

description: _____

SPIRITUAL ACTIVITY

description: _____

FOOD CHOICES DAY ❻

Breakfast: _____
Lunch: _____
Dinner: _____
Snacks: _____

PHYSICAL ACTIVITY steps/miles/minutes: _____

description: _____

SPIRITUAL ACTIVITY

description: _____

FOOD CHOICES DAY ❼

Breakfast: _____
Lunch: _____
Dinner: _____
Snacks: _____

PHYSICAL ACTIVITY steps/miles/minutes: _____

description: _____

SPIRITUAL ACTIVITY

description: _____

LIVE IT TRACKER

Name: _____

Date: _____ Week #: _____

My activity goal for next week:
○ None ○ <30 min/day ○ 30-60 min/day

loss/gain _____ Calorie Range: _____

My week at a glance:
○ Great ○ So-so ○ Not so great

My food goal for next week: _____
_____

Activity level:
○ None ○ <30 min/day ○ 30-60 min/day

RECOMMENDED DAILY AMOUNT OF FOOD FROM EACH GROUP

GROUP	DAILY CALORIES							
	1300-1400	1500-1600	1700-1800	1900-2000	2100-2200	2300-2400	2500-2600	2700-2800
Fruits	1.5 – 2 c.	1.5 – 2 c.	1.5 – 2 c.	2 – 2.5 c.	2 – 2.5 c.	2.5 – 3.5 c.	3.5 – 4.5 c.	3.5 – 4.5 c.
Vegetables	1.5 – 2 c.	2 – 2.5 c.	2.5 – 3 c.	2.5 – 3 c.	3 – 3.5 c.	3.5 – 4.5 c.	4.5 – 5 c.	4.5 – 5 c.
Grains	5 oz eq.	5-6 oz eq.	6-7 oz eq.	6-7 oz eq.	7-8 oz eq.	8-9 oz eq.	9-10 oz eq.	10-11 oz eq.
Dairy	2-3 c.	3 c.	3 c.	3 c.	3 c.	3 c.	3 c.	3 c.
Protein	4 oz eq.	5 oz eq.	5-5.5 oz eq.	5.5-6.5 oz eq.	6.5-7 oz eq.	7-7.5 oz eq.	7-7.5 oz eq.	7.5-8 oz eq.
Healthy Oils & Other Fats	4 tsp.	5 tsp.	5 tsp.	6 tsp.	6 tsp.	7 tsp.	8 tsp.	8 tsp.
Water & Super Beverages*	Women: 9 c. Men: 13 c.	Women: 9 c. Men: 13 c.	Women: 9 c. Men: 13 c.	Women: 9 c. Men: 13 c.	Women: 9 c. Men: 13 c.	Women: 9 c. Men: 13 c.	Women: 9 c. Men: 13 c.	Women: 9 c. Men: 13 c.

*May count up to 3 cups caffeinated tea or coffee toward goal

DAILY FOOD GROUP TRACKER

GROUP	FRUITS	VEGETABLES	GRAINS	PROTEIN	DAIRY	HEALTHY OILS & OTHER FATS	WATER & SUPER BEVERAGES
1 Estimate Total							
2 Estimate Total							
3 Estimate Total							
4 Estimate Total							
5 Estimate Total							
6 Estimate Total							
7 Estimate Total							

FOOD CHOICES   DAY ❶

Breakfast: _____
Lunch: _____
Dinner: _____
Snacks: _____

PHYSICAL ACTIVITY   steps/miles/minutes: _____

description: _____

SPIRITUAL ACTIVITY

description: _____

FOOD CHOICES — DAY ❷

Breakfast: _____
Lunch: _____
Dinner: _____
Snacks: _____

PHYSICAL ACTIVITY — steps/miles/minutes:
description: _____

SPIRITUAL ACTIVITY
description: _____

FOOD CHOICES — DAY ❸

Breakfast: _____
Lunch: _____
Dinner: _____
Snacks: _____

PHYSICAL ACTIVITY — steps/miles/minutes:
description: _____

SPIRITUAL ACTIVITY
description: _____

FOOD CHOICES — DAY ❹

Breakfast: _____
Lunch: _____
Dinner: _____
Snacks: _____

PHYSICAL ACTIVITY — steps/miles/minutes:
description: _____

SPIRITUAL ACTIVITY
description: _____

FOOD CHOICES — DAY ❺

Breakfast: _____
Lunch: _____
Dinner: _____
Snacks: _____

PHYSICAL ACTIVITY — steps/miles/minutes:
description: _____

SPIRITUAL ACTIVITY
description: _____

FOOD CHOICES — DAY ❻

Breakfast: _____
Lunch: _____
Dinner: _____
Snacks: _____

PHYSICAL ACTIVITY — steps/miles/minutes:
description: _____

SPIRITUAL ACTIVITY
description: _____

FOOD CHOICES — DAY ❼

Breakfast: _____
Lunch: _____
Dinner: _____
Snacks: _____

PHYSICAL ACTIVITY — steps/miles/minutes:
description: _____

SPIRITUAL ACTIVITY
description: _____

LIVE IT TRACKER

Name: _____

Date: _____ Week #: _____

My activity goal for next week:
○ None ○ <30 min/day ○ 30-60 min/day

loss/gain _____ Calorie Range: _____

My week at a glance:
○ Great ○ So-so ○ Not so great

My food goal for next week: _____
_____

Activity level:
○ None ○ <30 min/day ○ 30-60 min/day

RECOMMENDED DAILY AMOUNT OF FOOD FROM EACH GROUP

GROUP	DAILY CALORIES							
....	1300-1400	1500-1600	1700-1800	1900-2000	2100-2200	2300-2400	2500-2600	2700-2800
Fruits	1.5 – 2 c.	1.5 – 2 c.	1.5 – 2 c.	2 – 2.5 c.	2 – 2.5 c.	2.5 – 3.5 c.	3.5 – 4.5 c.	3.5 – 4.5 c.
Vegetables	1.5 – 2 c.	2 – 2.5 c.	2.5 – 3 c.	2.5 – 3 c.	3 – 3.5 c.	3.5 – 4.5 c.	4.5 – 5 c.	4.5 – 5 c.
Grains	5 oz eq.	5-6 oz eq.	6-7 oz eq.	6-7 oz eq.	7-8 oz eq.	8-9 oz eq.	9-10 oz eq.	10-11 oz eq.
Dairy	2-3 c.	3 c.	3 c.	3 c.	3 c.	3 c.	3 c.	3 c.
Protein	4 oz eq.	5 oz eq.	5-5.5 oz eq.	5.5-6.5 oz eq.	6.5-7 oz eq.	7-7.5 oz eq.	7-7.5 oz eq.	7.5-8 oz eq.
Healthy Oils & Other Fats	4 tsp.	5 tsp.	5 tsp.	6 tsp.	6 tsp.	7 tsp.	8 tsp.	8 tsp.
Water & Super Beverages*	Women: 9 c. Men: 13 c.	Women: 9 c. Men: 13 c.	Women: 9 c. Men: 13 c.	Women: 9 c. Men: 13 c.	Women: 9 c. Men: 13 c.	Women: 9 c. Men: 13 c.	Women: 9 c. Men: 13 c.	Women: 9 c. Men: 13 c.

*May count up to 3 cups caffeinated tea or coffee toward goal

DAILY FOOD GROUP TRACKER

GROUP	FRUITS	VEGETABLES	GRAINS	PROTEIN	DAIRY	HEALTHY OILS & OTHER FATS	WATER & SUPER BEVERAGES
1 Estimate Total							
2 Estimate Total							
3 Estimate Total							
4 Estimate Total							
5 Estimate Total							
6 Estimate Total							
7 Estimate Total							

FOOD CHOICES   DAY 1

Breakfast: _____
Lunch: _____
Dinner: _____
Snacks: _____

PHYSICAL ACTIVITY   steps/miles/minutes: _____

description: _____
_____

SPIRITUAL ACTIVITY

description: _____
_____

FOOD CHOICES   DAY ❷

Breakfast: _____
Lunch: _____
Dinner: _____
Snacks: _____

PHYSICAL ACTIVITY   steps/miles/minutes: _____ | ### SPIRITUAL ACTIVITY

description: _____ | description: _____
_____ | _____

FOOD CHOICES   DAY ❸

Breakfast: _____
Lunch: _____
Dinner: _____
Snacks: _____

PHYSICAL ACTIVITY   steps/miles/minutes: _____ | ### SPIRITUAL ACTIVITY

description: _____ | description: _____
_____ | _____

FOOD CHOICES   DAY ❹

Breakfast: _____
Lunch: _____
Dinner: _____
Snacks: _____

PHYSICAL ACTIVITY   steps/miles/minutes: _____ | ### SPIRITUAL ACTIVITY

description: _____ | description: _____
_____ | _____

FOOD CHOICES   DAY ❺

Breakfast: _____
Lunch: _____
Dinner: _____
Snacks: _____

PHYSICAL ACTIVITY   steps/miles/minutes: _____ | ### SPIRITUAL ACTIVITY

description: _____ | description: _____
_____ | _____

FOOD CHOICES   DAY ❻

Breakfast: _____
Lunch: _____
Dinner: _____
Snacks: _____

PHYSICAL ACTIVITY   steps/miles/minutes: _____ | ### SPIRITUAL ACTIVITY

description: _____ | description: _____
_____ | _____

FOOD CHOICES   DAY ❼

Breakfast: _____
Lunch: _____
Dinner: _____
Snacks: _____

PHYSICAL ACTIVITY   steps/miles/minutes: _____ | ### SPIRITUAL ACTIVITY

description: _____ | description: _____
_____ | _____

100-MILE CLUB

WALKING			
slowly, 2 mph	30 min =	156 cal =	1 mile
moderately, 3 mph	20 min =	156 cal =	1 mile
very briskly, 4 mph	15 min =	156 cal =	1 mile
speed walking	10 min =	156 cal =	1 mile
up stairs	13 min =	159 cal =	1 mile
RUNNING / JOGGING			
•••	10 min =	156 cal =	1 mile
CYCLE OUTDOORS			
slowly, < 10 mph	20 min =	156 cal =	1 mile
light effort, 10-12 mph	12 min =	156 cal =	1 mile
moderate effort, 12-14 mph	10 min =	156 cal =	1 mile
vigorous effort, 14-16 mph	7.5 min =	156 cal =	1 mile
very fast, 16-19 mph	6.5 min =	152 cal =	1 mile
SPORTS ACTIVITIES			
playing tennis (singles)	10 min =	156 cal =	1 mile
swimming			
light to moderate effort	11 min =	152 cal =	1 mile
fast, vigorous effort	7.5 min =	156 cal =	1 mile
softball	15 min =	156 cal =	1 mile
golf	20 min =	156 cal =	1 mile
rollerblading	6.5 min =	152 cal =	1 mile
ice skating	11 min =	152 cal =	1 mile
jumping rope	7.5 min =	156 cal =	1 mile
basketball	12 min =	156 cal =	1 mile
soccer (casual)	15 min =	159 min =	1 mile
AROUND THE HOUSE			
mowing grass	22 min =	156 cal =	1 mile
mopping, sweeping, vacuuming	19.5 min =	155 cal =	1 mile
cooking	40 min =	160 cal =	1 mile
gardening	19 min =	156 cal =	1 mile
housework (general)	35 min =	156 cal =	1 mile

AROUND THE HOUSE			
ironing	45 min =	153 cal =	1 mile
raking leaves	25 min =	150 cal =	1 mile
washing car	23 min =	156 cal =	1 mile
washing dishes	45 min =	153 cal =	1 mile
AT THE GYM			
stair machine	8.5 min =	155 cal =	1 mile
stationary bike			
slowly, 10 mph	30 min =	156 cal =	1 mile
moderately, 10-13 mph	15 min =	156 cal =	1 mile
vigorously, 13-16 mph	7.5 min =	156 cal =	1 mile
briskly, 16-19 mph	6.5 min =	156 cal =	1 mile
elliptical trainer	12 min =	156 cal =	1 mile
weight machines (vigorously)	13 min =	152 cal =	1 mile
aerobics			
low impact	15 min =	156 cal =	1 mile
high impact	12 min =	156 cal =	1 mile
water	20 min =	156 cal =	1 mile
pilates	15 min =	156 cal =	1 mile
raquetball (casual)	15 min =	156 cal =	1 mile
stretching exercises	25 min =	150 cal =	1 mile
weight lifting (also works for weight machines used moderately or gently)	30 min =	156 cal =	1 mile
FAMILY LEISURE			
playing piano	37 min =	155 cal =	1 mile
jumping rope	10 min =	152 cal =	1 mile
skating (moderate)	20 min =	152 cal =	1 mile
swimming			
moderate	17 min =	156 cal =	1 mile
vigorous	10 min =	148 cal =	1 mile
table tennis	25 min =	150 cal =	1 mile
walk / run / play with kids	25 min =	150 cal =	1 mile

Let's Count Our Miles!

Color each circle to represent a mile you've completed.
Watch your progress to that 100 mile marker!

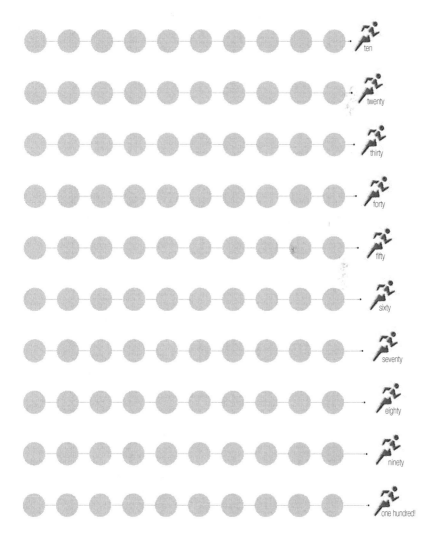

Made in the USA
Columbia, SC
08 September 2024